Phoenix Rising Yoga Therapy

PHOENIX RISING YOGA THERAPY

A Bridge from Body to Soul

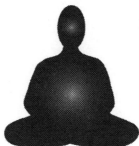

Michael Lee

Health Communications, Inc.
Deerfield Beach, Florida
www.hci-online.com

Library of Congress Cataloging-in-Publication Data

Lee, Michael, M.A.
    Phoenix Rising yoga therapy : a bridge from body to soul / Michael Lee.
      p.   cm.
    ISBN 1-55874-513-0 (pbk.)
    1. Yoga, Hatha. 2. Mind and body therapies. I. Title.
    RA781.7.L44 1997
    291.4'36—dc21   97-29358
                                          CIP

©1997 Michael Lee
ISBN 1-55874-513-0

Publisher: Health Communications, Inc.
          3201 S.W. 15th Street
          Deerfield Beach, Florida 33442-8190

Cover design by Andrea Perrine Brower

Thanks to Lee Shinefield, Nancy Nowak, Karen Hasskarl, Becky McFarland, Lori Bashour, and all practicing Phoenix Rising Yoga therapists for their commitment and support in taking this work to the world.

I dedicate this book to all of my teachers throughout my life, especially my wife, Lori and my daughter Keiron, my sons Christopher, Joshua, and Jack, and my mother and my father. I also dedicate it to all of my students, many of whom have also been my greatest teachers.

Contents

Introduction

The phoenix is a mythical bird of great beauty, fabled to have burned itself on a funeral pyre. In its state of destruction, one glowing ember remains in the fire that consumes it, signifying eternal life. It is from this place of immortality that new life evolves. The phoenix then reappears, transformed, rising out of the ashes of the fire with newfound youth and vitality, to live yet another cycle of life. That moment near death with only one ember remaining may well be the moment to which Patanjali was referring when, thousands of years ago he wrote the first yoga Sutra which says: "Now, the discipline of yoga!" Each of us may reach that moment when we begin in earnest, the quest for our spirit connection.

For thousands of years yoga has been a scientific approach to bring body, mind and spirit into harmony. Through the practice of yoga, I have learned that my body is a great port of entry to the inner state of my being, my awareness, my feelings, my mind, my truth and my soul. How to use it as such and how to support others in doing so has been my work for more than a decade. My quest has led me to discover ways to use my body, not only to gain knowledge and awareness but also to make changes in my life. By answering the call of my spirit, these changes are both desirable and in harmony with my *dharma*. My work has been to make these processes also available for others.

In doing this, I have realized that there are three very important elements in one's spirit quest. Firstly, like everything in creation, each one of us is unique with our own path to follow. Secondly, each of us has all the answers within us to help us find our own path. Thirdly, what I learned through my own journey was that even though I was using my body as a vehicle to my spiritual being, my passage to it was greatly enhanced by a loving presence, not a punishing one. With these elements in mind, I developed a modality that would facilitate a journey toward the discovery of one's unique being and honor its uniqueness in a way that would be more inviting than threatening. I have named this work Phoenix Rising Yoga Therapy.

The story of the phoenix has helped me through times in my life when I needed to be reassured that I would fly again. These periods usually occur when I feel vulnerable, alone and insecure after I have been though the fires of destruction, when some old belief, habit or way of being becomes obsolete and no longer a part of who I am. What has been is gone, what is yet to be has not begun and I am at the crossroads of transformation. These times preceding great change can be difficult for us or they can simply be a time for us to experience a new way of being. During this time of letting go of the old and embracing the new I have learned to use my body to fully experience all that is happening in each moment. I've also learned to accept what is happening, to listen deeply to a place inside and surrender to it. Then, and only then, am I guided to a course of action or a way of being. It is not unlike the practices of connecting to nature and the earth spirits used as ways of attunement by Native Americans and other ancient cultures.

As a symbol of transformation, the phoenix gives me the courage to embrace such change. She lets me know that I can endure the fire of transformation to a new, more desirable state of being and fly again. As German philosopher Georg Wilhelm Friedrich Hegel states in the *Philosophy of History*, "Spirit . . . does not merely rise rejuvenescent from the ashes of its previous form: it comes forth exhalted, glorified, a purer spirit." Because I believe this, I am drawn to look into aspects of my life to determine if I might be holding on to old ways just for the sake of being comfortable or because of the fear of change. If I am willing to enter the fire and be present to such awareness, a more exhalted state of being awaits me.

Although I am on a spirit journey, I have made mistakes. Sometimes big ones. Most likely, I will make more mistakes but hopefully not the same ones. Sometimes these mistakes have hurt others. For that I am deeply sorry for it has never been my intention to hurt or to harm. Yet I don't believe that we can hold ourselves or another to a promise of being perfect. Even though we aspire to learn and grow, imperfections will continue to arise. All I can do is sincerely commit to learn from whatever I encounter along the way. Like stones in a stream that are smoothed over the years by the flowing torrent, I will dwell in the stream of life and invite it to smooth my rough edges.

I wrote this book to serve as inspiration and understanding for those of you who want to learn to fly into, and through, the fires of transformation offered by life itself and for you who want to find your true nature by being present to your daily fears and joys—and in this process to be born into who you *are* and to die to who you *have* been. Your body is a valuable tool in this self-discovery process; in this book you will learn how to use it more effectively as such.

In the following pages I'll tell you about this process of discovering your Truth and learning from your body. The examples will come from my own experience and that of my colleagues and friends and my yoga therapy clients and students.* My wish is that by reading this book, you might find inspiration for your own journey; ways to support it through the practices of yoga; the desire to celebrate your unique passage in this life; and, that you will find hope and the possibility for transformation in everything that life brings to you, even when that seems impossible. Welcome to the ride.

*The names of clients in the case studies presented in this book have been changed to protect their privacy.

1

Now

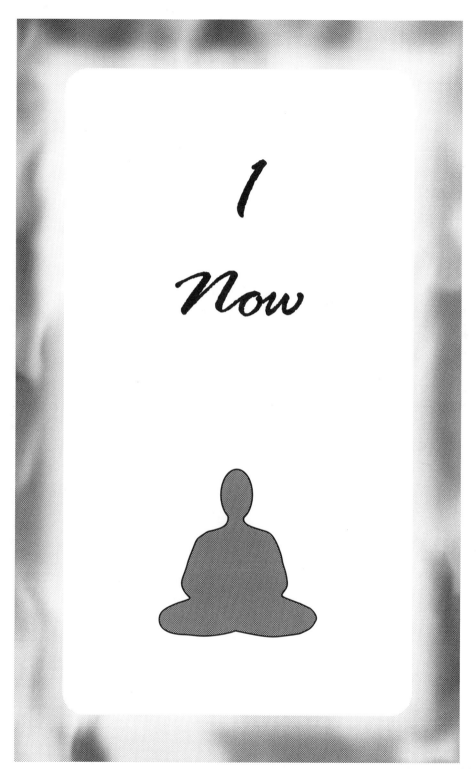

*W*hile developing and practicing Phoenix Rising Yoga Therapy, I've witnessed many people rise up from the ashes of their past to create a new future. I've seen people get in touch with a deeper self—that self who reflects their inner wisdom. I've seen them become aware of the hidden, unconscious aspects of themselves that color their perceptions and influence everything they do. The deep physical, emotional and spiritual shifts these people endure during yoga therapy give them the courage to face their intense and self-limiting fears and thus affect lasting and profound changes in their lives. Some clients have changed careers and addresses, ended destructive relationships and self-destructive behaviors. Some have pulled up roots and moved on; essentially realigning their lives to reflect the truths at the core of their being that were revealed to them during the yoga therapy.

Regardless of all the personal testimonies that validated and qualified the substance of this work, there was still a part of me that asked, "What is this all about?" and "What purpose does it serve?" These questions persisted, unanswered, until years later when I was a staff teacher at Omega Institute's annual program at Maho Bay on St. John, in the U.S. Virgin Islands. Another staff member of that program was Pat Rodegast, a well-known speaker, channel and author of several books including *A Manual for Living Comfortably in the Cosmos* (1985), *Emmanuel's Book* (1987) and *Emmanuel's Book II: The Choice for Love* (1989). Over the years, Pat and I had been faculty colleagues but had never worked with one another on a professional basis apart from attending one another's classes on St. John each year. So I was delighted when she asked to receive a Phoenix Rising Yoga Therapy session. We met one morning in one of the little tent cabins at Maho Bay after liberally applying bug repellent and setting the fan to keep the tropical conditions as pleasant as possible. Pat appreciated her experience and I enjoyed working with someone so deeply in touch with her spirit. After the session, she offered to pay me or give something in return. I asked for a private session with Emmanuel, not knowing that she very rarely gave them. She agreed and the following morning we set a time. I was excited and thought, *Ah ha! This is my opportunity to seek the answers to those questions that have been alluding me for years. Foremost: "Why am I doing this work? Why me? Why this? Why now?"*

After Pat went into meditation and connected with Emmanuel, I questioned the spirit guide about the purpose of my work. As I heard Emmanuel's response, an eerie feeling stirred in me and I was moved to tears.

> *We live in a time when many people are awakening. These human beings are starting to realize ways of living from a much deeper, spiritual place. They know the presence of the Divine within themselves. It requires incredible courage not only to face, but to embrace the monumental fear connected with moving in the direction of living from a place of attunement with the Truth. It's a bold move, strewn with obstacles challenging each seeker to disengage from the familiar in order to realize the Divine potentials that lie dormant within.*
>
> *In your own way, you've already traveled down this path of self-knowledge. You know what it's like. Some of those now working with you also have experience on this path. They, too, know the disturbance and turmoil, and ultimately, the sublime joy and liberation this process invites. It's important that you*

are available as a bridge, if you may, to others on their path. You and your work help others unite ordinary consciousness with an awareness of their inborn Divinity. More than your techniques, it is your loving presence that you offer that creates the safety necessary to cross the bridge.

The power of his words held me spellbound as I wiped away the tears. I believed what I heard and yet there was still the nagging voice within that sounded terrified by the implications of what I had heard. Upon reflection, the fear reached back to a prevailing Australian social taboo of being "too far out"; everyone is expected to be the same. Anyone who acts out of the ordinary, or who doesn't align with the expectations of their peers is liable to be confronted with disdain and disapproval. Simply put, most people are threatened by non-conformists, those perceived as different. The thought of my being a catalyst for people in their spiritual development was a little too far out for me to feel comfortable with it. Yet, I had been on my own spiritual journey long enough to know that the rainbow has many colors; that even if the trees in the forest look the same, each one is unique and beautifully different. I also knew I could not run from the truth I felt in my heart as I recalled Emmanuel's words again and again. In that moment, I surrendered my self-doubt to commit to my sacred unfolding through yoga and the bodymind.

"Now the discipline of yoga!" It had become time to embrace the ancient practices and begin the search for something more in life. What did the ancient sage, Patanjali, mean and how do we get started?

When Patanjali wrote those words, I am sure his definition of yoga was very different from what most people in the Western world today think of when they use the term. To many, yoga, and particularly *hatha* yoga, denotes physical discipline, often difficult to perform and not really connected to everyday life other than possibly being a good antidote for stress. So, to begin, I want you to know that when I address yoga in this book, I am doing so from a much broader perspective than the mainstream view and I hope more aligned with what Patanjali may have had in mind. (Yoga is a complete science, with the potential of making significant changes in our whole being, not just our bodies. It has the power to affect our feeling state, our total awareness of our selves, and ultimately our understanding of our connection to all that is.) There are some basic premises upon which yoga is based.

Firstly, everything we have ever needed to know as human beings is within us all the time. We have infinite wisdom. Now that's a way-out thought and if you don't immediately buy it, don't worry. You are in the company of 99 percent of the population. Just for a moment, consider that there might be some truth to it. Basically, we don't believe it to be true because we have never really experienced it as so. We get in our own way of knowing it mostly because we don't know how to access it. (I believe that we can use our body as our teacher to access our inner wisdom.)

There is a time and a place during each of our lives to seek out our teachers. As we learn our lessons, we need the teacher less and we begin to live our lives accepting growth and change. I have learned that by tuning in to the body we are able to learn a process. Later we can follow the same process without the body. We become aware, we accept and fully feel what is occurring in our life, and when appropriate we make the necessary changes, often with relative ease.

In many cases, to reach such a place, to even begin to tune in, requires a catalyst. Sometimes the catalyst is curiosity and sometimes it is despair. It can be that place where there is but one ember of hope left burning and something inside is calling us to expand our search for meaning.

As I examine my own life journey, I can say that this has been true for me. There came a time when it just seemed right for me to begin to study yoga. I had tried almost everything else the external world has to offer and was still coming up empty in terms of satisfying my spiritual hunger.

Satisfaction derived from worldly pursuits is temporal and incomplete at best, yet the path of our search is often paved with parties, alcohol, sex, success, power or anything else we might try to fill the void or sense of emptiness we feel. Yet we are, however, never quite able to quench our thirst. When we try to gratify our primordial hunger with substances, objects or pleasures, we are eventually led to the conclusion that there must be a better way.

I have returned to that place of knowing several times in my life. I believe I arrived there for the first time at around the age of 35 after having tried many dead-end paths to satisfaction. On the surface, I had a great life. I was married and had a comfortable home, wonderful and healthy children, a career with excellent possibilities, and most of the material possessions that I deemed necessary. My mind told me I should be happy. And although there were times when I was happy, I still longed for greater fulfillment.

I had explored the external world with great passion. I had traveled extensively and studied a wide range of subjects, experimented with different behaviors, lifestyles and experiences, engaged in politics to attempt to save the earth, lived in communal households, and read voraciously to satisfy my intellectual hunger. I still sought another way. I'd heard about people who were taking a more inward journey and became fascinated by the possibility of doing so myself.

It was when I was at one of the rocky crossroads of life that I began my practice of yoga which in turn opened a whole new window of reality for me. I'd been working as an organization development consultant for several years in Australia, leading team building workshops and personal- and organizational-growth experiences for management groups. I was fascinated by the powerful changes that occurred for people as a result of their deeper and honest levels of communication. I was also aware that the changes seemed to be somewhat superficial and short term. Although the strategies and

techniques I shared with these groups were received as both revealing and inspirational, it was often only a matter of time before
behaviors reverted back to the old familiar styles, particularly in
crises. It was difficult to teach people new coping mechanisms that
endured when the world around them continued to be "business as
usual." I became frustrated at first, and later somewhat despairing in
knowing that what I was doing may not be making that much of a
difference.

I had expanded my personal-growth vocabulary by attending a
wide variety of alternative and New Age workshops in the early
'70s. I became adept at New Age jargon and approaches. I confidently confronted, shared, and could "get off it" with relative ease.
And yet I was still the same old "new me" after the exhilarating
effects of the workshops and seminars wore off.

I sensed there had to be more to transformation after observing
how I still withheld a part of myself from life in general as well as
from many people around me. My protective stance shielded me
from being too vulnerable among my colleagues in the corporate
world as well as at home with my wife and family. In many ways, I
lived a very private life on the inside. No one really knew me, not
even my family. I had been confronted in some workshops and had
briefly touched moments of deeper truth, but that certainly wasn't a
place from which I lived my day to day life.

This awareness created the inner conflict necessary to motivate
me to find answers to what was stirring in my soul. I became
intrigued by the transformational prospects yoga offered to the
awakening process as I listened to my friend Ted, a retired Catholic
priest and an impassioned world traveler, relate tales of his wander-
ings throughout India in search of himself and Truth. There was a
stirring deep inside me as he spoke of sitting at the feet of Sai Baba
and listening to yogic wisdom. I was fascinated by the possibility
that wisdom resides within each one of us—that we really *are* Divine
beings. Although I believed him intellectually I did not have any

experience on which to substantiate my belief. His journey also seemed just a little too strange for me to fully integrate. I also had trouble accepting that all we need to do is find a way to let this internal knowing—this inner truth—express itself. At the same time, my interest was ignited to learn more about this simple approach to life that brings about unity, harmony and enlightenment as it embraces all religions and all people.

I began to read yogic texts and practiced *hatha* yoga postures daily by following the book *Richard Hittleman's Yoga: 28 Day Exercise Plan*. At first it seemed the traditional *hatha* yoga postures held little value, and I had great difficulty concentrating, coordinating the breath and putting my body into challenging, unusual positions. I maintained my inspiration to keep practicing by trying to convince the members of my communal household that these practices of Hindu origin were neither weird nor evil, but were instead the work of the Divine. Within a few months, I began noticing change—not only physical changes to my body, but emotional and psychological shifts as well. Day after day, as I listened to my body, followed its energy flow and observed sensory impressions and feelings, my understanding of who I *had* become and who I *might* become took on new meaning. I felt a growing sense of compassion toward my housemates in their struggle to accept my practices and noticed that I wasn't as angry as I'd been. I was becoming much more content and accepting of life as it *was*, and not as attached to my concepts of how I thought it *should* be. I began to look forward to my yoga practice and found it easier to concentrate and to be absorbed in the moment. As an antidote to the stress in my life there was no argument that these practices worked. There also seemed to be the possibility of even more.

The uncomfortable part was that I was beginning to know more about myself. I began to see my imperfections more clearly and the ways I unconsciously avoided living from my heart. Many years later as a professional yoga therapist and teacher, I have seen this process repeat many times with my students. My yoga practice was creating the possibility of real and lasting change. Simultaneously, fear, uncertainty and desire struggled within me. Not knowing what else to do to continue, I sought support and guidance from those more experienced on this path.

I began to frequent the local yoga community with visits to the Siddha Meditation Center and the Satyananda Ashram and also attended a one-day workshop with Swami Satchidananda when he came to Australia. I was impressed by the beauty and simplicity of this yogic path. There was an absence of righteousness and dogma. There was also a sense of humor around the level of consciousness and spiritual condition of the human species. My newfound companions and I sought to discover ourselves with compassion. I would often arise at five in the morning to go to the nearby Satyananda ashram to practice yoga before going to work. I would leave there feeling a deep sense of joy and fulfillment in my whole being as I drove down to the city through the beautiful Adelaide hills. I even considered living in India for awhile to more fully immerse myself, but decided that I didn't have to experience a foreign culture to find my spirit, even though the yoga practices were born in India's culture. I also realized that many traditional yoga masters had moved to the United States and were developing ways to integrate yoga into Western culture. To my Australian eyes, the United States was a country that represented the best and the worst of everything in the world—a country of extremes—and I recognized that if there is to be a planet-wide spiritual awakening, the possibility of it emerging in America was great. The still quiet, but rapidly growing, voice within me knew I wanted to be a part of that and that I would find what I was looking for in the United States.

In 1982, I traveled to a diverse number of yoga centers and New Age communities throughout America where I encountered many interpretations and expressions of the spiritual life. My path was strewn with paradox and disillusionment. Although many people I met aspired to lead truly spiritual lives in tune with their higher selves, there were indications that the political and material aspects of their communal lives were not always in harmony with the spiritual. I saw signs of repression, dogmatism, material excess, poverty bordering on malnutrition and often good intentions unmanifest through poor organization.

At the same time I found places that on some level gave me the experiences I was seeking. One of my most significant experiences occurred at Ananda ashram in the Sierra Nevada foothills of California. During one pre-dawn meditation, I experienced, for the first time, energy flowing through my body in rhythmic waves. My practice of meditation created the pinnacle from which I observed my mind in action, and I felt sensations of release and exhilarating freedom throughout my entire being during daily yoga practices. Along with these feelings of expansion and liberation, I experienced the intense feelings of vulnerability that accompany a deepening awareness of oneself. I felt raw and open as I allowed myself to experience a broader spectrum of life. When I left the insulating sanctity of Ananda, my perceptions had shifted and I was much more sensitive to everything around me. My instincts seemed sharpened and finely tuned; my senses heightened. Reality was shiny and new like a freshly washed window. I heard even the faintest sounds, felt changes in temperatures, and was acutely aware of people and objects nearby. In several instances, I felt I had the ability to anticipate what was going to happen next. It took several days on the road, including a period of incubation in a friend's apartment in Los Angeles before I felt ready to be in the world again.

I asked myself if I might not be better off spending more of my life in the seclusion of an ashram. Surely it seemed safer if I was to practice this path. My life for the next several years was to embrace both courses and this was to be an ongoing question for me to ponder. Several years later, it had become apparent to me that my life was to be in the world. My quest was the pursuit of the truth within—

within me, within each one of us and in *all* things—that resonated
with what my heart already knew. It was also clear that yoga was the
one discipline of all I'd explored that felt in harmony with this. I
desired to practice and teach yoga, but I wanted to do it in a way
that allowed me to remain in the world, not hidden away from it.

Eventually I returned to Australia to research available avenues to
satisfy my desire for growth. My intent was to find a teacher and a
community where my family and I could temporarily reside that
would provide a sanctuary in which to take my yoga practice and
inner quest to a deeper level. The proverb "When the student is
ready the teacher appears" tells exactly what happened next.

Soon after my return, I was introduced to a woman from the
United States who knew of a heart-centered spiritual community in
Pennsylvania whose residents were followers of Bapuji, Swami
Kripalvandaji, and his disciple Yogi Amrit Desai. She lent me a
video entitled *The Path of Love*, which showed Bapuji receiving
flowers as he descended the steps of a quaint cottage in a forest, and
that convinced me that this was the community I was looking for. I
was drawn by this man's gentle radiance and his serene, loving facial
expressions, as well as those of his followers. What I didn't know was
that he had died a year earlier and that the community, known as
the Kripalu Center for Yoga and Health, was in the process of moving from Pennsylvania to the Berkshires in Massachusetts. I received
welcoming and encouraging responses to my inquiries about residing
there, took a year's leave from my job in Australia, and prepared
myself, my wife, and our two children to live and study there.

I took an independent masters degree program through Vermont
College which gave me the opportunity to live at Kripalu and use
my residency as the focus of a thesis on the therapeutic value of yoga
using myself as the subject. I immediately fell in love with my new
abode, the environment and the people. I drew much needed inspiration for my spiritual journey from the practices, the interactions,
and the evening gatherings with senior residents and Amrit Desai.

My thought was that perhaps this was a community I could live in for a long time. The hardships of a confined living space, and family adjustments to our new dwellings seemed insignificant now that my life felt on track. Even the discomfort of diving inward to confront myself was welcome. My self-concept went into immediate turmoil and revolt, however, when I was assigned to work on the maintenance crew. All my conditioned beliefs about myself emerged. My ego constantly insisted I wasn't good at working with my hands. My adopted script decreed I was supposed to be a teacher and I struggled fiercely with resistance as I tried to keep my familiar identity intact.

The longer I held the posture of living in the energy that prevailed at Kripalu at that time—the more layers I was able to shed from the casing of my ego-mind. It was humbling, empowering and challenging to live in a community where the inhabitants shared the intention to live from love and, certainly to me at that time, they appeared to do so very well. Yoga and meditation were the core of our daily discipline and spiritual practice.

Soon, I was assigned to the staff where I assisted with and then taught a variety of programs including: Introductory Yoga Weekends, Yoga Teacher's Training, Raw Juice Fasting and Holistic Health Education. I also continued to work on my graduate studies. In my teaching I was developing a capacity to engage in, and lead, body-oriented experiences that would promote deep inner work. There were times when I and other residents would assist and support each other in yoga postures using a variety of props to enhance what was emerging naturally in the body. It was during one of these sessions that I experienced an unforgettable event that changed my life.

One of my friends was using a wall to support me in the triangle posture on my right side when my body began to quiver uncontrollably. I witnessed an intense red-blue, burning sensation in my right hip and believed I had pressed into the posture as deeply as I could, feeling pain that wasn't really pain. My mind was shouting, "Get out of here! Stop now! What are you doing? Get on with it." I was definitely at an edge between the known and safe and the unknown, unsafe territories of bodily experience. The escalating sensations in my right hip were becoming almost unbearable when my attention shifted from what was happening in my body to what was taking place in my attitude. I was becoming more and more agitated and wanted to release out of the posture. Placing his hand gently against my chest, my friend embraced my growing resistance by encouraging me to stay in the pose a while longer. His affirming presence made me feel safe and I surrendered again and again into what was happening in the moment, deepening my breath and simply witnessing the strange noises emanating from my mouth and throat. The hot, fire-red burning seemed to pour out of my hip like a volcanic eruption. My whole body vibrated and I felt warm tears streaming down my face without my knowing why. My body began to feel very small as I re-experienced myself as an eight-year-old boy standing on a school playground about to be beaten up by a group of older boys. The terror of that frightened child penetrated every cell of my being as I continued to release emotionally, feeling out of control, yet totally safe in the memory my body was releasing to consciousness.

Incredulously, the sensations passed almost as easily as they had come and I came out of the posture feeling very different. Internally, I felt stiller, quieter, suspended in a sense of timelessness. I was very *present*—to the moment and to myself. My friend stayed with me a while continuing to give his gift of unconditional acceptance of what I was experiencing that had helped me to surrender into the experience as deeply as I had. I sensed he had the same kind of trust in the natural wisdom of the body to support healing that I was experiencing.

Afterwards, I journaled about what had happened using the same kind of questions I'd been trained to ask others during my days as an organizational development consultant.

These following questions have been known to reveal deeper levels of truth:

- What really happened?
- What did I feel?
- What is the significance of this experience?
- How does this affect my life?
- What aspects of this experience show up in other areas of my life?
- In what situations, and when, have I felt this fearful before?

While reflecting, I realized I'd been living my life in fear of what "big people" might do to me, probably since I was eight years old. A "big person" was usually a male in a position of power or authority who could use his status to affect my life. Whether or not these authority figures were actual threats didn't matter, I perceived them as being capable of influencing me in ways that were destructive and coercive. I reacted to the imaginary threat by staying away from "big people" or humoring them to protect myself from harm. I vowed to never let these tyrants get to know the real me, particularly the part that was afraid. This defensive coping strategy manifested in a sense of helplessness that had persisted into adulthood. I truly believed I would never have the strength needed to stand up to people in positions of power and authority. I channeled my anger about my helplessness by confining assertive behavior towards people of my own stature and engaging in overt and covert political activity to work against the "big people."

With this new awareness, I realized how ridiculous it was for me to continue this pattern. Physically, since I had released all these pent-up memories and emotions from my musculature, I felt three inches taller and safe for the first time—no longer was I afraid to fully inhabit my body. I walked with greater ease and moved more confidently. Within a few weeks I was making friends with some of the "big people" in the Kripalu community. I was in awe of the power of my physical body to effect emotional and psychological change. I began to focus my energy to work on this primal, intuitive level of body-centered transformation and integration, eventually evolving into the work that is now called Phoenix Rising Yoga Therapy.

In the ensuing years, I developed a repertoire of assisted yoga postures and dialogue techniques to support clients in releasing physical tension which was often connected to some kind of emotional, mental, or spiritual release. The idea was to support the client in holding a yoga posture at "the edge"—a place of not too much stretch but not too little either. Then with coaching to focus the client's awareness on their unique experience, the client would be invited into dialogue around what they were experiencing in regard to body sensations, thoughts and feelings.

My experiences working with clients in this manner were as varied as the clients themselves. The one common thread running through all the experiences was that each person was somehow affected by the work and would have a different experience of themselves after our session together. For some, awareness occurred primarily at the physical level. These people usually felt freer, softer and more flexible as their bodies released long-held tensions during the posture assists. Others were affected more on the emotional level as feelings of anger, shame, fear and joy were expressed by crying, shrieking or laughing. Many shared a sense of spiritual realignment which resulted in an awareness of and deeper connection to their inner being and sense of expanded self.

It became apparent to me that this approach to yoga had the ability to tap into unconscious memories of past experience that in some way had been stored in the body. When brought to awareness, these memories revealed aspects of a person's core belief system which was usually formed in early childhood and maintained through adulthood. It was not possible to anticipate what would happen or what would be uncovered during a session. The more invisible and unobtrusive I was, the more clients felt they had permission to surrender to their body's innate wisdom to express itself as energy, awareness, thoughts, feelings and sensations. The process unfolded naturally, guided by their inner being as I simply provided a space of acceptance and love, affirming all aspects of each person as the work of the Divine within.

As my yoga therapy practice with clients evolved, I worked part-time at the nearby Desisto school—a special boarding school for adolescents with emotionally based behavior issues. Most of the students were from professional families, very aware, open to new ideas and often very intelligent. The school was highly innovative, under the guidance of its founder Michael Desisto, a man I greatly admired and who was to become a friend and supporter of my work. The school program utilized Gestalt therapy techniques and sessions within the context of a supportive organizational structure. The results of introducing the therapeutic yoga techniques I was developing within this educational environment were both encouraging and impressive. Several of the therapists working with the students commented favorably on the impact of the yoga work I was doing with them. After receiving a session or class, students often opened up and were more inclined to share their whole story rather than just the chosen bits and pieces. Students were also more willing to access the emotional realm rather than stay in a mind space. These encouraging results gave me the needed confidence to continue to practice and develop my yoga-based work. My work here was also intended to provide me with a bridge from the seclusion of the ashram into the world.

My two older children were teenagers and unhappy with some aspects of living in the residential community. They craved the freedom of living in a regular household with TV and having their friends visit. Suddenly I was faced with the task of deciding how to make this transition into the world again in a way that supported my work and fulfilled the financial and material needs of my family. The courageous, uninhibited part of myself was enthusiastic about continuing my work as a yoga therapist and sharing and expanding upon the exciting discoveries I was making. The scared part warned, "Quit messing around with this stuff and get a real job," while the confident part assured me, "You can do anything you really want to do. Just put yourself to it." The battle between the inner voices persisted, but eventually the confident one held sway.

We moved from Kripalu to nearby Stockbridge. My clientele grew gradually as I extended my business beyond the small Berkshire towns to include New York City. Ten clients grew to twenty, and the larger my clientele became, the more I believed I was really doing something worthwhile. But, I *still* had doubts. I questioned whether I was living in pretense; whether my clients were being honest with me about the value the work imparted in their lives. Perhaps the changes my clients were experiencing would have happened anyway. Even though I wasn't sure where the work would end, I was enjoying it and felt inspired enough to continue.

Soon, several clients encouraged me to teach them what I was doing, so they too could create transformative experiences for others. Thus, the first Phoenix Rising Yoga Therapy training program was born. In 1987, seven people registered for our first six-day program held in Trenton, New Jersey. In reflection, I admire those pioneers. I knew very little, in terms of detail, about the work. I knew how to do the work but not how to teach it. Our inexperience forged a remarkable program, in that we taught each other as we went along. Most importantly, everyone was affected by the cocreated process of using the body as a doorway to the soul.

Exercise

FOCUS ON PHYSICAL SENSATIONS

Do you recall a time in your life when you have been inspired to look more deeply within yourself? If so, how did you choose to do that? Have you ever tried using your body as a vehicle for deeper self-awareness?

Try now to sit quietly for a few moments and focus your attention on your experience of your physical body. Simply become a witness to your experience without trying to judge or label any aspect of it. Continue this practice for five minutes if you are able. Then reflect on your experience. What did focusing on your body create for you? What sensations did you notice? Did you notice any particular thoughts or feelings?

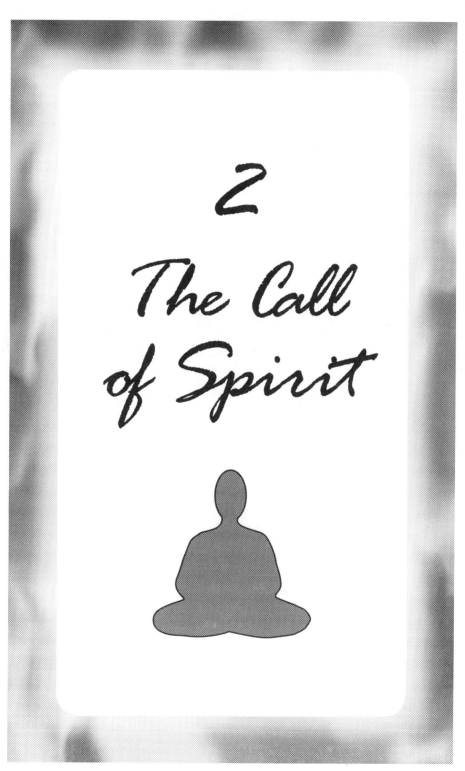

2

The Call
of Spirit

*W*e live in a time when spirituality is no longer a hidden part of life or just the domain of established religions. The practice of yoga—the oldest of all spiritual pursuits known to us, and all it offers, is being rediscovered and developed in many new directions. The growing emphasis on the inclusion of the body in contemporary psychotherapy practice, and the explosion in interest and enrollment in yoga classes around the country are signs that yoga is once again emerging as a path to be followed. I delight in playing a part in that development, and am particularly interested in an approach to yoga therapy that focuses on empowerment of every aspect of one's being.

I believe that an empowered being is one who is strong in spirit, able to attune to a deeper level of knowing and then live from that place. This person is clear in mind and able to choose wisely from a world of many choices. To do this, one must fully feel their emotions and use them creatively as a source of learning and growth. To live fully requires living in a body that is connected to these spiritual, mental and emotional aspects of being human.

For the past 20 years, I feel I've been crossing a bridge. What I have left behind is a way of life that appeared to be working but at a deeper level was spiritually incomplete. My early life was more about making the right moves than recognizing or living out the unique call of my soul. The act of being present enough to one's self to hear the message from inside is sometimes referred to by yogis as one's *dharma.* Each of us hears a different message. Once I understood that I needed to listen to my inner guidance, my task became not only to do that for myself, but also to help others do the same. I call the process I created to do this, Phoenix Rising Yoga Therapy.

Despite the ease with which I became aware of the need to be true to my purpose, putting it into practice was more difficult. For instance, I knew that I was supposed to be teaching about living one's Truth, but at the time I was in a nine-to-five job that did not allow for this. I was being called to shift from something secure and comfortable to something unknown and uncertain. Many mornings on my yoga mat followed by long conversations with my friend Ted—who didn't give me answers to my questions but simply stayed quiet and listened to me so I could hear myself—helped me to make that move. He was the witness I needed.

I needed guidance to support me through a process of witnessing. I wanted a catalyst for my own learning instead of just a source for answers. This process illuminates the spirit within us, yet allows us the freedom to discover ourselves. It requires an inner stillness which the body can provide. We need to attune to our inner voice and listen with our whole being rather than just our mind. We can then integrate what is revealed to us by having someone be our witness. We are then ready to take the next step.

Phoenix Rising Yoga Therapy uses the body and breath as doorways to the spirit. Non-directive verbal processes support reflection and integration, so that what is revealed by spirit is brought to action in life. We all have access to information about ourselves, much of which we don't even know exists. The process of transformation requires that we trust sufficiently to enter this unknown domain.

My early experiences with yoga therapy were based on a more traditional approach. The therapist had the knowledge; the student didn't. The therapist prescribed; the student followed. The focus was on symptoms and naming what is broken or defective. A particular result was expected, and that was that something troublesome would be fixed. The therapist could learn the required techniques by focusing on doing and knowing what to do.

The thinking inherent in that paradigm has been the mainstay of our society for many generations because our focus has been on achieving definable results. We have not discarded it because it continues to serve us well. If I have a problem, know what it is and want it fixed, this is the path I will most likely choose. It works well and has a valid place in our world.

The process of transformation requires a different paradigm. At some point in our spiritual growth, we need to take the leap into trusting ourselves to know our own answers. We learn this by being supported by approaches that take us to the edge of our knowing and beyond. We have to be familiar with ways of being present to life that preclude compliance or dependence on others, or experts for the answer. (Our therapies must teach us to know and trust ourselves.)

In the following case study a woman allows herself to answer her call to spirit by using this approach.

Martha said she'd heard of Phoenix Rising Yoga Therapy from a friend. She was particularly inspired by her friend's newfound *"joie de vivre"* since coming to see me. During our preliminary conversation, Martha told me that although she appeared to be content on the surface, she was really not happy most of the time. She wanted more satisfaction in her life. I told her that we would be using her body as the vehicle for her growth; and, it would guide us to explore whatever was presented. I told her that she was in charge of the session, that she could call on me at any time to change what we were doing and that I would respect her wishes.

I asked Martha to close her eyes as I supported her into the first posture, an assisted version of *bhujangasana* (cobra pose), which I chose because I had noticed that as we spoke, Martha held her hands across her chest from time to time. I helped her to focus her awareness on her whole body and breath, feelings, sensations, images, and thoughts and to notice what she was experiencing. When I asked her what was happening, her first response was, "This is hard!"

I shifted into being with her experience and responded, "So you are finding this hard. Tell me about that."

"I don't want to be here in my body. I want to run away like I always do."

"Run away?"

"Yes, leave my body and go somewhere else, daydream, watch TV, eat—anything to not be here in this damned body."

"So you want to run away and not be in this damned body. Tell me more about that."

"It's like a scared feeling. When I begin to notice and feel my body, I get scared."

"When you begin to notice your body you get scared."

"Uggggggh. Yuk!"

"Yuk?"

"Yes, this is very hard to do. The feeling of wanting to run is very strong."

Martha was demonstrating a capacity to be present to her body, despite the difficulty, despite the resistance. I stayed with her and affirmed her willingness to be with what was happening. Then I asked her to go a step further. I asked her to exaggerate the feelings and sensations she was experiencing and to tell me what was happening.

"Oh my God!" she exclaimed. "This is so weird!"

"Weird?"

"Yes. After I exaggerated the feelings, they went away and then I began to feel and see myself as a young woman about 20 years ago."

"Tell me about that."

"Well, I was rather pretty, actually. Not fat like I am now. I was standing in a field and felt very free. I didn't need anybody, I was feeling my power as a growing and independent woman."

"A growing and independent woman?"

She didn't say more but began to cry. I stayed with her and when she finished I eased her out of the posture. She then told me her story.

When Martha was about 20 she began dating a young man whom her parents and friends considered an "eligible" partner. At first she thought so too, but as the relationship progressed she had her doubts. She liked him, but something didn't feel right. She dismissed it as her fear of commitment and marriage. When he proposed, she cast aside her doubts and went ahead with the marriage, much to everyone's delight. She adapted to married life, including moving to an unfamiliar city where her husband's company had transferred him. Her first child was born and for awhile the joy of motherhood fulfilled her; but deep down she felt empty. She began gaining weight, but dismissed it as her body's response to childbirth. After her second child was born she gained even more. Around this time, she began to dislike her body and herself.

I listened, occasionally repeating what I heard. From time to time, I searched my mind for some gem of wisdom for Martha. I resisted the temptation to speak and brought myself back to simply being with her.

While telling her story, Martha said that she realized how she had sold out on her desire to be an independent woman when she married. She said that, at times, she had dreams that reminded her of that part of herself that longed to be an independent woman, but never paid much attention to them.

She paused and sighed when she'd finished her story. I asked her what she'd done that helped her reconnect with this part of herself. She said her willingness to be present to herself in her body, even when she felt like running, was the most compelling element. She was also aware that by going into the uncomfortable sensations, she was passing beyond them.

Martha's question now was, "Will I have to leave my husband? I don't think I want to because, even though it's been hard for me at times, I do really love him."

"What do I do?" she implored.

I asked Martha to close her eyes and then I guided her into meditation. I asked her to go to a place inside her that was beyond the confusion, a place that loved her, accepted her, and only wanted to serve her. When she felt comfortable there, I suggested that she ask for guidance, wait for it and then tell me about it.

She opened her eyes and spoke. "I don't have to make any decisions right away. I need to trust my body and learn more from it; connect with it again. Get to know myself and my 'independent woman,' and trust that we will find a way to express ourselves together as we get more comfortable with each other."

I could not help feeling in awe of her wisdom as she spoke, marveling yet again at the way her body supported the expression of her inner truth. Here I was enjoying her process and wanting to insert some of my own insights and I caught myself. It was difficult for me to be purely a witness and stay out of the way.

I saw Martha for several more sessions and then maintained contact with her over the following year. She did not leave her husband. As she began to let her "independent woman" speak and to play and work in the world more, her husband's love and admiration for her were rekindled. She began to sing again and was offered a solo part in a local summer production. She lost weight without dieting (her previously preferred approach) after further guidance from her Higher Self in another one of our sessions. In all our sessions my approach was similar. I trusted that by supporting Martha in opening to herself through her body she would find what she needed. My job was to support her, but to stay out of the way.

This is relatively simple, but not always easy. My Western mind is often eager to leap in to supply the answer. When I could stay out of the way, she could often get in touch with her inner guru. This, I believe, was facilitated by the release of energy that had long been held in check in her body. It did not surprise me that she could observe her own willingness to face her discomfort.

(I have seen it many times and I believe it is one of the profound ways in which the body supports the process of deeper awareness on *all* levels of being. So often we run away from our uncomfortable sensations and never allow them to teach us. If we confront them, they often dissipate and take us somewhere new, often into deeper levels of awareness. Chaos may ensue for a while because we are being called to a new way of being. Note, however, that in the meditation, not only did Martha receive inner guidance about what she needed to do, but even how to go about following it.

Martha also experienced a spiritual transformation. She had lived much of her life as a compromise, doing what seemed to be the right thing, and had denied her "independent woman" to please her family. Initially, she discovered this by being present to herself in her body. As she accessed her real power, she was able to express herself more fully. She was being drawn to follow the unique path that life was making available to her, and to find ways to reveal her uniqueness to the world—to follow her *dharma*, a call to spirit. Phoenix Rising Yoga Therapy helps her along in this process by freeing the blocked energy in her body and allowing its expression. The result for Martha is that she experiences a deeper connection to her soul.

Each one of us has a unique and wonderful gift to give the world. Once we are in touch with who we are and allow our true nature to blossom, this gift is easier to give. We become able to share more of who we are as loving beings. For that to happen though, we must have the courage to be who we are, to attune to our unique spirit and allow its full expression through a process of waiting and witnessing. Only then can we take action, follow the openings that come, and face new fears that arise. Phoenix Rising Yoga Therapy is a practice that promotes transformation by drawing on the unique wisdom of the body. At the same time, for empowerment and transformation to occur, the process must honor the spirit and stay out of its way. When this happens, yoga is *therapy*.

3

Thank You, Body

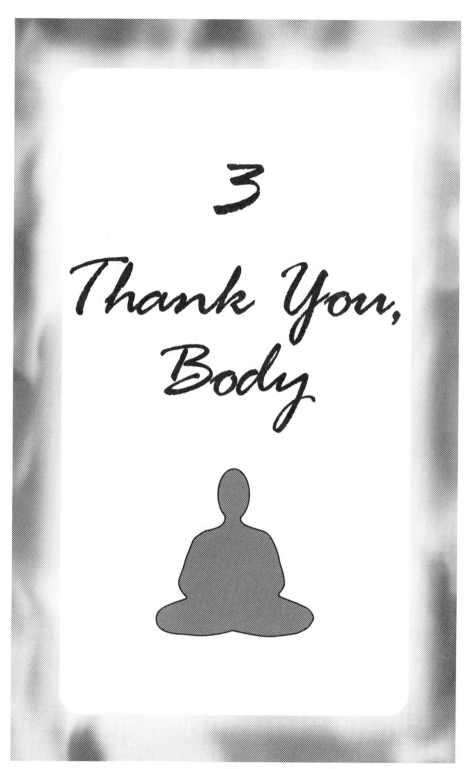

*H*ave you ever thought to look at your body in the mirror in the morning as you get out of bed and say, "Thank you, Body. Thank you for all the times you have adjusted and changed. Thank you for all the times you have healed. Thank you for dealing with all I have forced upon you. Thank you for being there for me in every moment of my life. Above all thank you for trying your best to keep me safe at all times."?

The last sentence may seem a little strange but I believe it is appropriate. Our body works very hard at keeping us safe. Before birth and right up until death, our body is one of our primary sources of protection. Often it keeps on working even when the rest of our being has given up. When we are under threat or attack, the body quickly mobilizes itself to resist or to run. No matter what the outcome of any traumatic experience we may have encountered, our body fought to protect us.

All of us have witnessed incredible changes in our lives. Advances in computer technology during the last decade have changed and continue to alter the way we live our daily lives. Many resist these changes based on the belief that they take us away from ourselves; that our lives become less personal and more machine oriented. Instead of going to a bank teller we now go to the ATM. Our conversation with the bank teller may have been limited but with the ATM there is no conversation at all unless it is with ourselves. This is just one area of our lives wherein we have less "connection" to people. Is this a problem? Do we need that connection? I have thought about these questions and come to the conclusion that we cannot turn back the clock. Why would we want to? There is much that our advances in technology have brought to us that is highly desirable. We have the capacity now to communicate globally. Barriers between nations and people are dissolving. We are at last beginning to take responsibility at a global level for the fragile ecological balance that supports life on our planet. My laptop, on which I write this manuscript, goes with me on trips and enables me to not only capture my thoughts but also to communicate them via modem to a vast electronic audience. Information on any subject is just keystrokes away on massive on-line databases. At the same time, we crave human connection. It is our connection with others that provides nourishment for our spirit. Through the loving presence of others we can reflect the essence of our soul back to ourselves. Without it, we wallow in the sea of illusion and ultimately the pain that stems from a mind that is not grounded in spirit.

In the early '80s, I was taking an extended "time-out" and living on the Greek island of Lesvos. As far as I knew, there weren't any psychotherapists on the island and I thought that was pretty strange. But people there generally seemed content with life. There was a guy with a big smile on his face riding his donkey, women sitting on the steps laughing and making pasta, shopkeepers enjoying their customers, and people in the streets looking happy. What was going on here that was creating this level of contentment? Was it the sun? Maybe the religion and beliefs? I had nothing much to do for three months but to ponder questions such as these.

One morning I was having breakfast in the local tavern and one of the local guys who worked there was late. In fact, he was very late. He usually arrived way before me. He came in and I could understand enough of the Greek language to know what was going on.

It was a long, involved story. He was at his brother's place the night before. His brother was recently married and had started to fight with his wife. He was feeling very sad for his brother but he knew his brother was being stupid in the fight so he also felt compelled to take care of his brother's wife. On and on the story went for about 20 minutes. Amazingly, the whole time, his boss just listened, and at the end he hugged him and then they both began to work.

All the while, I'm thinking to myself, back home he'd have said something like, "My car wouldn't start" because he would have been too busy or too embarrassed to cover the whole story. His boss most certainly would not have listened for too long and as for giving him a hug—that is highly unlikely. And then I realized that's what it is. People on Lesvos tell the whole story and other people listen—they connect—that's the reason for this contentment. In our busy business lives we don't connect as much as we need to. In fact, we are so caught up in our heads that we don't even take the time for conversation beyond that which is related to getting things done. Over time, we lose "touch" even with that part of ourselves that needs to connect.

Although as you read this you may agree with what I am saying, there is another level to understanding this concept—the experiential level. Try moving and stretching your body for a few moments. Let your body bend to one side; as you do, take a full deep breath, letting the exhalation just fall out. Hold that position for a few seconds and continue to breathe. Notice what happens. If you can stay with it awhile and not push too hard, you may find that you begin to relax a little. You may even notice that your thoughts slow down. Your stillness may be difficult to stay with if you can obtain it at all. You may feel compelled to stop and get on with the next important thing in your life, dismissing the exercise as a waste of time. If you can be present to that, and anything else that comes to you, you may begin to learn something about yourself. In my work, I have found again and again, that clients very quickly "drop in" to a deeper level of experience of themselves when they are supported in using their body as way of getting "in touch." It is often after they have "dropped in" that stories, feelings, experiences, fears, and joys will be witnessed and dialogued. My clients are just like the Greek waiter in that they want to tell their story and be heard and accepted. They want that connection. By relaxing and telling their story or relating their inner experience of themselves, a transformation begins. Their growth is enhanced when they reach a level of letting go, a degree of self-acceptance, self-processing and adjustment to life's mystery. Is there anything special I have to do to support this process? Not really. It is certainly not about *doing*, but rather about *being*. What I offer is a loving presence on all levels of being; body, mind and spirit. When this is given to another human being, it is difficult for them not to feel touched. It does, however, require their participation in the process. If their resistance is too great they just won't be able to "drop in." What we offer to people with this process is a vehicle, first of all, to help them reach that deeper level within them, and to get in touch with, and acknowledge, the story. They can't share it if they don't know it's there. There is no need to do anything with it. We don't have to fix it. They don't have to make it go away. It's simply about listening without judging.

Even when our conscious mind has forgotten, our bodies remember our stories. They remember our pain, our joy, and our long-forgotten childhood fantasies and freedom of expression.

One way to let your body remember is to tune in to it just like you would tune a radio to a particular station. When you take time to tune in to each area in your body and just be totally present to it, you may find it has much to tell you.

Once when doing a body scan with a client, she began, through her body, to remember running and playing in a meadow of flowers, feeling the sun and wind on her body. She recalled how beautiful it was to experience herself and her body in this way and to feel the sense of freedom it gave her. As a successful businesswoman she had not made time for her body to feel in many years. The next weekend she went home to rediscover her meadow. The following week a real estate transaction she had been working on somehow fell into place. Reflecting on it, she recalled how in her meadow, even though it was raining, she had released herself from the struggle that had crept into her life. Her "little girl" had remembered to play more and not to take the busy part of life too seriously. She remembered to be less attached to the outcome and to enjoy the ride. She returned to New York, called her broker and withdrew her bid on the property she was pursuing. Within the next hour the broker called back and the property was hers for much less than her original bid. She had created what she wanted by letting go. Her body had re-educated her in that process that her mind had forgotten.

In a way, our body is a map. It was there with us during every significant event, feeling, trauma, and celebration. It was not a passive bystander, it was involved. It *responded* to what was happening just like the other parts of us responded. Sometimes, depending on the situation, its response was lasting. If it needed to act to protect us in some way, it may have continued to go on doing that long after the threat had disappeared. If our body experienced pleasure, it may have sought out that pleasure again and again, even long after it ceased to satisfy. Despite this, it did what worked at the time. Just as it would be inappropriate to use only a part of ourselves to engage in a competitive sporting event, it is also inappropriate to only use a part of ourselves to manage and understand our lives. Imagine a basketball coach instructing his team to play only as their bodies felt like it without a game strategy or without routine practices. In the same way, it is inappropriate to engage life with only our mind. It is a wonderful tool but it has its limitations. Our bodies also have limitations but they also possess a wealth of information about us if we take the time to "read" them and to "listen" to them. They are also a wonderful vehicle for supporting us in embracing ourselves in those aspects of being that get lost in our external world. In fact, our bodies are another doorway through which we gain access to ourselves. This is a particularly important doorway when we have effectively blocked the others through a compulsive focus on our external world.

So I often do thank my body. This morning as I thanked my body, I was reminded of Sarah's story.

I had been doing Phoenix Rising Yoga Therapy with Sarah weekly for about two months. She had come to see me after a week-long Rest and Renewal program at the Kripalu Center. It had been her first experience with yoga and she had been amazed to find that during some of the morning yoga sessions she'd become afraid and wanted to run away. She believed her body was opening up to something she wanted to investigate further. In several of our sessions she experienced the same feelings. Each time, Sarah was able to stay a little longer with the feelings that came up, but would then tighten her body and shut them off. From my years of experience with this process I'd learned to completely accept the wisdom of Sarah's body in choosing this response. There was no need to rush the process toward a particular outcome. I was just present to her and accepted whatever happened. Sarah also learned to do this and began to relax around her need to know.

One morning we chose to work with the assisted legs-to-sides posture. Sarah lay on her back while I gently raised one of her legs until she felt a stretch in her hamstrings. Then, for about 10 minutes, I carefully guided her leg out to the side of her body at a right angle, moving it toward the floor. This posture often taps into fear-based tension held in the thighs, hips and pelvic area. It also often evokes feelings of vulnerability so I always work slowly with it and usually only after trust is developed with the client and they are comfortable with this work. We found her "edge" in the posture and I helped her focus her awareness on the sensations, the feelings and her breath. Quickly she moved through the scared feelings and into a deep cathartic release. She screamed and sobbed for several minutes. I gave her space and encouraged her to experience the process. When the release subsided, we began to talk.

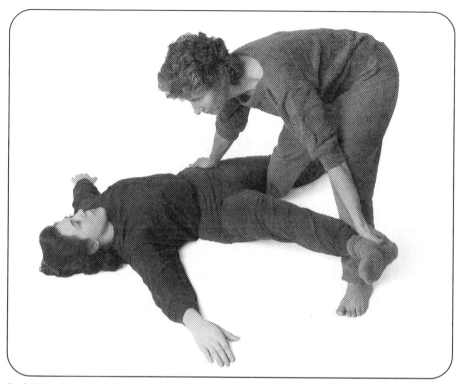

Stefi Shapiro and Becky McFarland demonstrate legs-to-sides posture.

Her story was very moving. She said she'd relived the experience of being molested for the first time at the age of seven. She knew that she had been abused as a child but had, until now, suppressed the details. It was difficult for her to share now but she would, time and again, wipe away the tears, take a deep breath and continue her story. She told of feeling intense "locking sensations" in both of her inner thighs. When she allowed herself to go into the feelings in her body and stay with them, the memories began to flash back. She saw herself as a little seven-year-old, with her little legs working so hard to protect herself. There was nothing any other part of her could do, but her thighs continued to resist throughout the experience. She also said that for her entire adult life, she has been unable to have satisfactory sexual relationships. Whenever the possibility arose, her thighs automatically locked up, just as they did when she was seven. But it was only then, years later, that she made the connection. She said that the first feelings she experienced with the awareness were anger. Anger at her uncle, anger towards all men, anger at me and anger with her body for locking up. Further on she noticed the anger subside, and as her thighs relaxed, she felt grateful for the release. She realized that she was able to obtain the release by accepting it. By following my guidance during the experience, to "Stay with the sensations. Let yourself into the sensation, into the feelings. Just be present to what is, without the need to do anything with it." When she did this, her body relaxed and she felt different than she had ever felt in her life. Her body had stopped fighting and she was safe. This had never happened before. Before she only felt the possibility of safety if her body was locking. She began to feel grateful for her body rather than blaming it. Her body had only been resisting because it was the only way it knew how to keep the little girl safe. The little girl had no other resources and did not know any other way to prevent such a violation. The 38-year-old woman had many more resources to keep herself and the little girl inside her safe from any harm. She could choose when to resist and when not to, rather than resisting as an automatic response to situations that triggered memories of the past. When she would notice her body resisting she could simply go with it with acceptance and love, and it would let go all by itself. Sarah was very excited about what she had learned from her body and how she could use it in the future to help heal her past wounds.

Sarah's story illustrates a dramatic and deep therapeutic way in which our bodies can serve us. There are other less dramatic ways, perhaps not so deep, but equally important.

More important than anything else, our bodies are our connection to our soul. As such, they offer us the opportunity to connect with the part of us that is beyond the human condition—the part of us that is Divine. Now you might ask that if we truly are Divine, why is it so hard to find that part of ourselves? Well, I believe that it's not that easy to be in touch with that part of ourselves. It can be downright scary. One of the first problems we face at a very young age is the problem of how to be present in our world—how to show up. We have to exist, and in order to exist we have to adapt to what is happening around us. Part of the human condition is that it necessitates being born into an imperfect world, a world that is often confusing, full of paradox, and full of people in the process of evolutionary transformation, not yet fully transformed or evolved. The individual adapts to survive in such an environment. A child is born in a state of perfect harmony with the universe. Innocence is lost as the child grows and adjusts to the temporal ways of being. The child then spends the remainder of life overcoming the split that this creates. "How absurd!" you might say. "Why is this necessary? Why not just spare the agony and not incarnate at all?" Well, I'm not sure of the reason or even if there is one. It's like asking why trees need to be trees. It does seem, though, that another process happens that goes deeper.

If our lives truly offer many opportunities for transformation, and we take those opportunities, we must, in the process, strengthen our soul. Maybe life is "finishing school" for our soul. Maybe in dealing with, and then releasing, all the fear we've created during our early adaptive processes, we become stronger in spirit and as a result we have more to give. We are then able to contribute to some kind of collective evolution in consciousness. By being strong trees we strengthen the forest. "So what!" you might say. If so, so be it. I cannot convince you that the transformational journey is worth embracing. No one convinced me, so why should I try to convince you? I embraced the journey, because my experiences suggested that it was a game worth playing. Many of those experiences came primarily through my body, but not exclusively. My deep body experiences in yoga have considerably helped me deal with transforming life experiences that do not come through the body but through

some other life event or circumstance. During the years I have been
practicing and teaching Phoenix Rising Yoga Therapy, I have, time
and again, seen people come to the same conclusion. Their body
opens them to an experience of themselves that is very much about
connecting to spirit. As a result they *know* there is more. In some
ways it seems an addictive process. You get a taste and you want
more. The "inner journey" has begun. How does this happen?

I believe we are present as both human and Divine at all times.
We tend to get lost in the human and we tend to "forget" the Divine.
When we take our attention inward and stay focused there for a
time, we reconnect. It's that simple. For centuries spiritual masters
have taught practices and techniques to accomplish this. Phoenix
Rising Yoga Therapy is a collection of some of these, combined with
others from more recent times. As we enter the body with great
awareness, supported by another's loving presence, focused on our
breath and willing to let go, we enter another domain of being—the
domain of spirit. Even during brief demonstrations of the work,
people go to a place of great tranquility and say afterwards that
they'd felt deeply connected to the "core" of their being. So then
what could be scary about that?

Sometimes when you do connect in a deep way to your spirit, you
become painfully aware of the "opportunity"—the extent to which
you are not daily living in harmony with that spiritual knowing. In
Phoenix Rising work we even have a part of the integration process
that is used for that purpose—to bring to focus the "opportunity."
Some like to interpret opportunity as deficit and punish themselves
for having it. If you do that, then it's natural that you might resist
visiting those places that might bring this into focus. Also, when
you get to uncover an opportunity, it usually means you have to do
something with it. That means work or at the very least you may
have to adapt to some kind of change. If you prefer that your life has
some degree of continuity to it, change can be threatening.

One of the reasons why so many established and orthodox religions tend to attack New Age transformational therapies is because transformation may occur. Transformation means change, and it means getting in touch with a unique version of the "Truth"—our very own. That notion is very unsettling to people with a vested interest in teaching "the one true path." Interestingly enough though, it was rebellion against this dogmatism that motivated Martin Luther to break established tradition in the 16th century. We find history full of similar events. It seems that at some level we know that our Divinity is within us, but as soon as we get a handle on it, we want to make it true for everyone else by institutionalizing it. Maybe the old adage "a little knowledge is a dangerous thing" is applicable to the transformational process. Once we begin the journey and become aware of our Divinity, we need to be extra careful not to try to wrap it up and interpret it for everyone else. The drive to do this is likely motivated by the fear that we might not quite have it right but if enough other people see it in the same way we will feel more secure in our new knowledge. And the truth is that no two people ever see or experience the same thing in exactly the same way. Each experience is unique unto itself. That concept can be either downright scary or totally beautiful. It all depends on your level of trust in the Divine.

Exercise

THE BODY SCAN

The body scan is best done with eyes closed, so have someone read the following directions to you slowly while you follow along in your body.

Stand in a comfortable position.

During this experience I am going to guide you as we go to, and around, different parts of your body. Simply allow yourself to go there without judgment. There is no need to understand it, no need to explain it and not even a need to change it or shift it. In fact it is better if you don't. Simply notice what's there and we will move on.

Begin by taking your awareness to your feet. Eyes closed and breathing easy, notice where the weight is distributed on your feet at this time; whether it is more on the front, the back, the inside or the outside. There is no right or wrong location; it just is where it is.

Now take your awareness to your ankles, and notice which parts of your ankles are working most to support your body at this time.

Come up a little higher to your calf muscles and notice anything that is happening there.

And then a little higher to your knees. Notice if your knees are holding your body up from a locked or an unlocked position. Again there is no right or wrong; just what you experience—that's all.

Bring your attention to your thighs: inside, outside, front and back. Notice which part of your thighs is working to hold your body upright at this time. Where is the work coming from in your thigh muscles?

Come up a little higher still—to your pelvis. I'd like you to imagine that your pelvis is like a bowl of water. The bottom of the bowl is your groin, the top of the bowl is your waist and the bowl is filled to the very brim. Notice which way the water is likely to spill out of the bowl. Is it likely to come out the front, or the back or maybe the side? Simply notice. In other words, which way is your pelvis tipping? Is it tipping down at the front, down at the back, or over to one side or a combination? Again, there is no need to make any adjustment or corrections. Just simply notice the way it is.

Taking the awareness to your abdominal region, notice

any areas of softness or hardness, any areas of more sensation or less sensation.

Come to your solar plexus, your rib cage, your chest. As you breathe, notice where the breath goes and what happens to your solar plexus, your rib cage and your chest. Notice any areas where the breath goes very easily, and any areas where the breath tends to get stuck and doesn't want to flow.

Move your awareness up to your shoulders and notice your shoulders in relation to your chest and the rest of your body. Do your shoulders want to come forward? Do they want to go backward or do they want to rise up out of your chest? Do they want to drop away from it? How do your shoulders want to rest in relation to your chest? Just simply notice.

Notice your arms in relation to your shoulders, and your arms in relation to the rest of your body. Do your arms want to come forward or go back? If you were to give your arms freedom of movement, in which direction would they want to go? Simply notice.

Come back up your arms to your shoulders; to your neck. Notice which part of your neck is working to support your head.

Bring your awareness to your head. If your head were given freedom to move, in which direction would your head want to go? Would it be forward, backward, to one side or the other? Are there any other parts of your body that want to go with your head in any direction?

Now notice your whole body—your whole body from your feet all the way through to the top of your head. Notice which parts of your body want to come forward, and which parts of your body would prefer to go backward. Is there any conflict between the two parts that would like to come forward and the parts that would like to go backward? If there is a conflict, notice where it occurs in your body.

Focus again on your whole body. This time notice the texture, the feel, the sensations and maybe even the colors or the shapes you experience within your body. Ask yourself who lives here in this body right now. "Who is home here right now?" Then take a breath and let it all go.

Take another breath and let it go. Now, before you take your attention from your body, do one final thing. Take a moment to thank it. Thank your body for all that it has done. Thank it for all the places it has been. Thank it for all the adjusting it has done. All the times it has kept you safe; all the times it has healed. "Thank you body, thank you body."

Open your eyes and find a place to sit quietly. Take a few moments to reflect on the tour you took around your body. What did you discover? Did any awareness come to you that may be connected to your life in some way? Is there something you can learn about yourself from this? What is it?

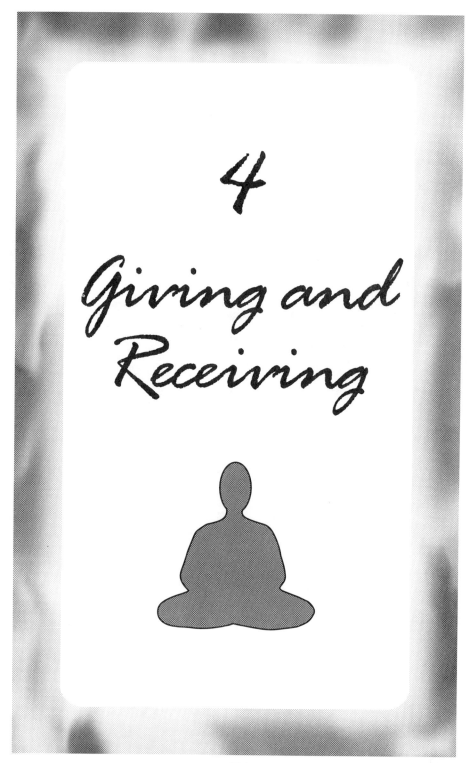

4

Giving and Receiving

I have learned that for me to feel fully alive, I need to be giving and receiving love. It is the very process of life itself.

Giving and receiving are like night and day—you need one to have the other. You need one to understand the other. You need one to balance the other. That is a natural law. When we live in harmony with the natural law, our giving and our receiving are in balance. Sometimes one might exceed the other, but the seasons balance it all out. Does this mean we need an accountant to make sure we are getting the right balance? Not likely. If our lives are in balance, it happens naturally. Furthermore, there is no effort to it. I recall Amrit Desai's words, "Does a flower make an effort to spread its fragrance?" Of course not. It is an effortless happening. So, too, is giving and receiving love. There are many barriers to the balancing though and they all come from concepts that attempt to defy the natural way of being. They often show up with great clarity when we explore them with our bodies.

During a workshop, after a partner exchange of assisted postures, I invited participants to share their experiences. Ellen said that she experienced difficulty when receiving but felt great while giving.

"Tell me more," I implored.

"Well, I just couldn't relax."

"You couldn't relax?"

"No, I kept wanting to see if she was okay. I was afraid I would be a burden for her."

"You were afraid of being a burden?"

"Yes. I didn't want her to feel uncomfortable trying to move my body around."

"So what if she was?"

"That would be terrible."

"Terrible?"

"Yes. I've *never* been able to let myself be a burden for anyone!"

"Not for anyone? Ever?"

"Well not really. A few times I've had to lean on my husband when I've been ill but it was worse than being ill."

"So receiving was difficult but you really felt good giving to your partner?"

"Sure. That part was easy. I could see that she was going deep into her experience and that I was helping her and that felt great."

"So it feels great to give?"

"Yes, I've always felt that way ever since I can remember—even as a little girl."

"Even as a little girl?"

"Yes, I remember whenever I took care of someone my mom would smile at me and tell me how wonderful I was."

"How about when you received a treat?"

"Oh no! I would always have to share it with my little brothers and sisters so they wouldn't feel jealous. Wow! Isn't that amazing? I couldn't let myself receive even then."

"You are surprised by that awareness?"

"Yes. It makes so much sense though. As soon as I begin to just totally receive, my body does this weird thing, like gets all fidgety and can't relax. Just like when I was a little girl and every time I got something given to me. I'd always have to make sure that no one else was upset or having a hard time with it."

I suggested to Ellen that she ask her partner how she had experienced the exchange. Her partner was surprised that Ellen was worried about her. She said she found Ellen easy to work with, not a burden, and enjoyed giving to her. She had noticed her fidgeting but just stayed present without judging it, as we had been teaching her. Ellen was surprised. "So it was just my imagination that I was being a burden—my ongoing story about myself."

I verbally recognized Ellen's willingness to be open to these new awarenesses and validated her generous nature. The part of life that is about empathy and taking care of others, was a part of life she had mastered. Anytime she wanted she could easily be this way. She didn't consider it wrong to act this way. It only became a problem for her when this was the *only* way she could be, and when it prevented her ability to receive when she really wanted to receive, as in the exercise she had just participated in. For her, the learning edge was in choosing when to receive and when to give and how to feel great about both. When that could happen, her whole being would be more in harmony with the so-called natural law of giving and receiving and her life would flow more easily. I suggested to Ellen that she might want to explore this more with her body; that the next time she received and felt that fidgety feeling, she might choose to let it happen, to go into it and hang out with it. She agreed to try that, and after the next exchange she offered to share her experience.

"Now I'm even more amazed," she began.

"More amazed?"

"Yes. As you suggested, I watched for the fidgety feeling. At first it wasn't there, but then after a while it started to happen. Instead of freaking out and trying to take care of my partner, I just let myself feel the urge to want to do it. It was like riding a wave. I had to really focus to stay with it. Almost like a contraction in childbirth. Feeling the pain and not struggling with it. Then I began to see or imagine this big hole and I was being whooshed through it. On the other side there was this beautiful blue light, very soft and calming. I was just floating around in it. I have never felt so relaxed. I don't even know how long I was gone but I remember feeling my partner's hand on my forehead and how great it felt and how I could just let it be there and feel the love coming through."

"So you could let yourself receive the love?"

"Yes, yes! I really could and it was great."

"Ellen, I think it's important that you reflect again on exactly what you did that made that possible. Tell me what you think that was."

"Well, I focused on the uncomfortable feelings I was having without either reacting to them or trying to push them away. I just let them be there. I guess I accepted what was happening to me even though I didn't like it all that much."

"So acceptance played a big part?"

"Yes."

"What else?"

"Another thing was that I followed along with what happened next. I let myself into the experience more fully even though I didn't know what was going to happen. But you know there was something else happening too. I was beginning to trust my partner giving to me and it was by doing that that I was able to go deeper. Her loving presence was like a wand waving and saying, 'Come on in—it's okay,' and I trusted it."

"So you were already letting yourself receive the loving presence of your partner and felt safe to go into unknown places."

"Yes."

I reminded Ellen about the feelings she experienced in her whole being when she was finally able to let go. "Your body now has a new experience to reinforce your learning. It won't forget and it will help remind you in future situations, when the fidgeting comes along, that you have a choice. You can, at that moment, choose to either give in to the fidgeting and take care of the person giving to you or you can go into the sensations and choose to receive. I suggest you don't think about one choice as good and one as bad—just think about it like choosing between apples or oranges. Either choice is okay depending on your preference." Ellen was glowing and ecstatic about the possibilities that were now awaiting her in many aspects of her life.

After Ellen graduated from our Phoenix Rising Yoga Therapist Training Program it was no surprise that she soon attracted several clients who had similar stories to hers, who had imbalances in their giving and receiving. I asked Ellen how it was for her to work with people like herself in this regard. "Great!" she exclaimed. "Several times a week I get to see myself mirrored back to me and each of my clients teaches me something new about myself as well as learning something about themselves. It's like we are all doing this dance together. Life is so much richer since I began to accept myself as someone who is a work in progress and just let myself be open to whatever comes along. I'm really receiving much more than I could have ever imagined. The absolutely amazing thing is that the more I receive the more I have to give and the more I want to give."

Ellen reminded me of that natural law of the universe: *When I am able to fully receive, then am I able to fully give*. A lot of folks mistake receiving as taking too much or being greedy. There is a subtle but important difference. (Receiving is just letting in what's already there for you. Greediness is an effort to make more for yourself than you need and to try to get it away from someone else so you can have it. It's altogether different from receiving.) There is also a subtle and important difference between receiving and just waiting for the universe to give it all to you. I'm amazed by the vast number of Abundance workshops and books around these days that preach the idea that all you have to do is be "open to the universe" and you will receive all the abundance you need. While there is a half-truth to this, it is often oversimplified. Certainly the act of receiving does not need to be a struggle, so this part of it has some truth. (On the other hand, "God helps those who help themselves." Or, as the Arabs say, "Trust in Allah but don't forget to tie your camel.")

Ellen was able to receive because she could see what was in her way and how she could actually do certain things to let the universe give to her. In other words, she had a part to play. There was some learning that needed to be done. (We are not separate from the universe—we are the universe—and very much participants in the Divine order of things.) We have to do our piece in order to align with the universe. Now it does not have to be an effort or hard work—yet it requires our active participation.)

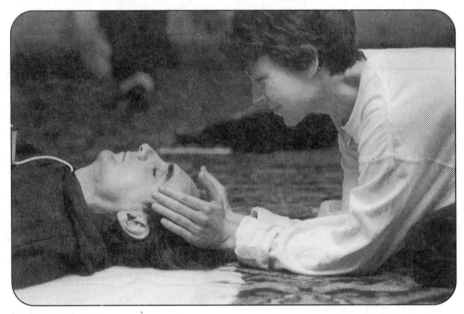

Loving presence

Giving can be just as much of a problem as receiving. For some, giving becomes an habitual set-up. I recall working with Rosa, a client for whom giving had become her way of being. She had learned from early childhood that people liked her when she gave. It was a way to get noticed and to be loved. So she gave a lot and it worked well for most of her life. Or at least it appeared to. There was a downside, however. It was very tiring to be giving so much. It was also very draining. A lot of her life-energy was outer-directed and other-directed so that she was forever struggling. In response to the question, "How are you doing today?" she would let out a huge sigh, put a pained expression on her face, and between several shallow breaths, respond with "Aaw, okay, I guess." Just making a living and meeting month-to-month financial commitments was a struggle. In one of her early sessions she began to cry. When we explored what was happening, she reported that it was difficult for her to receive. Just the very act of allowing me to move her body into and out of the postures, as occurs in the process of this work, was too much for her to receive. There was something about it that wasn't right. On further exploration, she discovered that for her there was no such thing as "unconditional love." She always gave in order to get. To receive without having to give raised the possibility of giving without having to receive. This concept did not match her experience of herself and was disturbing to her at first.

In a subsequent session in a chest-opening posture, a lot of other awarenesses began to surface as well. She realized that she had a pattern of choosing relationships in which she could be the "giver" and would get the things she wanted from the "receiver." When the unspoken trade did not materialize for some reason, she would often stand in harsh judgment of the "receiver." She noticed how often she used the terms "unfair" or "not fair" in her relationships. In time, those she perceived as being unfair to her, became the target of her passive anger. No one could ever complete the trade as she expected and she was often left with the feeling of being unfairly treated by those to whom she gave so much of herself. Unlike the flower spreading its fragrance effortlessly, her giving had become a manipulative act. In allowing it to become so, she had stepped out of balance with the universe and with her spirit.

After this session, she also became aware of how shallow her breathing seemed to be in normal day-to-day life. After another session, she noticed how deep and full her breath seemed to be becoming and while it felt good, it also felt strange to her. When we explored this phenomenon in relation to her life, a flash of awareness came to her. She was experiencing difficulty just receiving air from the universe. She held within her being and her body a deep and clear belief that it was not okay to receive.

The older she became, the more difficult it was for her to receive. The more unfulfilled trades she compiled, the more anger she stored in her body. Her body was beginning to feel it. She was overweight and often suffered with swollen ankles and aches and pains. Her heart was beginning to show signs of fatigue and most of her life was miserable. Her husband left her because he could no longer live with her passive hostility. She was now aware that her ability to receive without expectations was the key to her liberation. Her self-suggested homework was to walk outside each morning and in five minutes take 20 long, deep breaths of fresh air. As she breathed she affirmed how much there was in the universe for her to receive. She began to temper her compulsive conditional giving and began to give only in situations where she could do so without expectation. Giving was now a source of joy for her. She began to nurture herself with good food and took a week-long yoga retreat to help her reconnect with her body. She sought counseling to help her deal with her feelings surrounding the loss of her partner in life. When I last saw her she was exploring business ideas with the intention of finding a way of expressing herself more fully in life. This was something she had always wanted to do but never had the time because she had been so busy giving.

Exercise

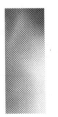

LEARNING TO GIVE AND TAKE

Find a place to sit quietly. Close your eyes and place your hands in your lap. Turn the left hand to face up and the right hand to face down. Begin to breathe deeply and feel the breath entering and leaving your body. Feel your body receiving breath as a gift from the universe. As you breathe out see yourself giving to the world around you. Bring your hands into focus as well, receiving through your upturned left hand and giving through your down-turned right hand.

Begin to notice the difference between the act of giving and the act of receiving. Notice how you experience your body in each mode. Notice any feelings. How do these relate to your life? Do any memories surface? Are you a better giver or receiver? How can you reach a balance?

5
The Edge

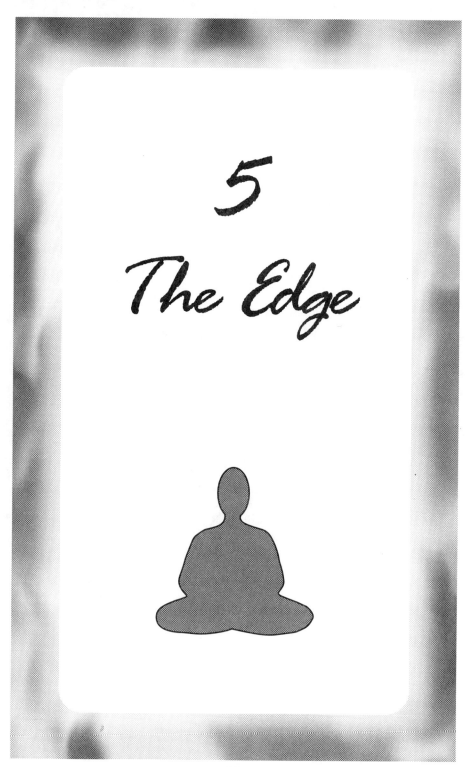

*W*hen I became interested in yoga I wanted to learn it all in 28 days as my first little book on the subject suggested.

As I began to try the various postures, I noticed how incredibly inflexible my body was. It would hurt a lot when I tried to place myself in the various positions described in the book. I began to doubt that yoga was really for me. Of course I had absolutely no idea of how to coordinate my body and my breath or how to use my awareness and focus it internally. So I experienced pain. I also knew nothing about "the edge," which I will soon explain. I bumbled along on my own for some time and did not give up. I began to practice the breathing exercises in the book and one day discovered the connection between the breath and the postures. When I used my breath to relax my body just as I was entering the threshold of discomfort in my body, my body would somehow open up a little more and it didn't seem to hurt so much. Later, I found I could actually focus my attention on the discomfort and just be present to it, rather than think about how painful it was and how I would never be a yogi, no matter how long I practiced these postures.

Later, I discovered what was probably the most significant single concept that was to open up my yoga practice and my life. It was the concept of "the edge." Shortly after I arrived at Kripalu, Yogi Desai initiated a system of morning *sadhana* (spiritual practice) for all residents of the ashram. A one-hour yoga routine (the same postures every day) was followed by a guided meditation, often led by Yogi Desai, and sometimes accompanied with chanting. I was committed to the morning practices and would make my way faithfully to the designated room for my group each morning at five o'clock. Some postures were held for a long time. It was during some of these longer periods when I experienced the most difficulty. I noticed that I could endure the pain of the postures that were held for a short time.

One morning, after a somewhat restless night, I found I was reaching intolerable levels of discomfort even when in the postures we were holding for only a short time. I found myself coming out of them ahead of the rest of the group and feeling very frustrated. I was trying to be willful and my willfulness was not working. It was clear to me that this was meant to be a willful practice. I was supposed to push a little to get in there and experience the discomfort. This was the only way I would progress physically and spiritually. At least that was what my mind was saying even though my body had a different story.

Luckily I was pragmatic enough that morning to conduct a little experiment with myself. I tried not trying so much. I let myself ease into the postures to a degree that I experienced only mild and tolerable discomfort. After doing this for a while I began to feel guilty. I was not doing my best. I was taking the easy way out. I felt terrible. So the experiment failed and I went back to trying again. My guilt gave way to the same old frustration, anger and pain.

Then I had a flash of inspiration: how about finding some feelings in between? Excited by this new possibility, I eased my body into the next posture and tentatively sought out that place in between. At first it was hard to find. I had to resist the tendency to try harder and then the temptation to back off too much. After practicing this a while, I began to find it and was soon holding postures at this new "edge." The results were amazing. I began to enter a state similar to what I had previously experienced only in meditation. I was able to become a witness to myself. I was able to feel the same uncomfortable, yet also inviting, feeling of entering a void. Then in the void, images, sensations and even new awareness would come to me. I was not the doer of the posture, I was the receiver. Within days my yoga practice began to take on a whole new meaning. It was at the edge that things really started to happen. At the end of each day's practice I would feel renewed. I began to connect with myself at a much deeper level. I became aware of things in my life that were in the way. One day I had an insight into my relationship with my children. I saw my fear of fatherhood. I let myself soften into being an inexperienced, sometimes insecure, but loving father. I did not need to be anything else. What exquisite liberation!

Later in the development of Phoenix Rising Yoga Therapy, I discovered that there was one thing better than being in a yoga posture at the edge. That was being in a yoga posture at the edge with someone else supporting me there. There was no effort even in holding and supporting the posture. I was free to give all of my attention to what was happening. The whole process became even more profound. Time and time again I have seen this happen with clients. Once they were able to enter and stay at their edge they often had experiences that were life changing. I became convinced that transformation happens at the edge.

Soon, I began to see amazing connections between the edge in yoga postures and the edge in life. Until I had discovered my edge and been able to accept it, I was forever striving for some conceptual result or goal. Once I'd accepted the edge, I learned that there was no need to get somewhere. Everything I needed to "get" was right here. That doesn't mean that I stopped setting goals and working to reach them. In fact, the more I accepted my edge the better able I was to achieve anything I set my mind to. I had learned to stop struggling. The process of striving to achieve something became simply choosing a direction and being with the experience moment-to-moment, making adjustments when appropriate. Had I not learned this valuable lesson I would never have created Phoenix Rising. Using my old pattern, I would have been far too willful for my own good, would have set unrealistic goals and then given up because they were unattainable.

On television I saw an interview with an ace jet fighter pilot who, in the face of extreme odds, had single-handedly taken on six enemy fighters and won. The interviewer asked him what he thought made a hero like himself. Was it a requirement to be a little crazy, or to have a disregard for life to be willing to put one's self at such extreme risk? The pilot responded that it was neither. To him it was about assessing a situation and knowing where the edge was. To him the edge was that place where he would certainly still be at risk but where, because of his honest self-assessment of the situation at hand, his own skills and the skills of his opponents, he would be able to take the risk with the odds slightly in his favor. It wasn't a question of bravado or heroism, but simply a fine-tuned awareness of what he was really facing. He knew where his edge was and he played from there.

You may find that success in every facet of life is based on the same thing. Unless you find your edge, there is no growth, no learning and no change. Too far back from the edge is boredom and atrophy. Too far out from the edge is self-destruction. Another discovery, both in the body and in life, is that the edge is always moving if we are willing to play it. It is always expanding into new unknown areas. Personally, as I learned to explore the edge in my body I learned to explore the edge in life. In the last eight years, in my forties, I have learned to ski cross-country and downhill, to create and give to the world a new body/mind therapy, to run a rapidly growing organization, to fly an airplane, to teach others how to teach, to marry again, to be a father twice more and to write this book. I have accomplished these things with relative ease. That same ease is available to all of us. You may discover that your ease can come from being as aware as you can of your edge in each and every moment, playing that edge and growing beyond it. My body and my yoga practice, and the focused awareness that came with it, taught me all about my edge. Integrating it within my life was the easy part.

Finding your edge requires a high level of presence. You can't find

it if your mind is somewhere else. This means that in your l
in your life) you have to be willing to go into and to be with what is
happening in the moment. You then have to be willing to stay there
long enough to tune into it and make the necessary adjustments.
This is really the process of transformation. It's the process of using
your awareness first and foremost—and then accepting what you've
found. It doesn't work to become aware and then go into denial or
self-flagellation. As a private pilot, I've read many aviation accident
reports, and I'm amazed at how many deaths have resulted from
denial—an unwillingness to accept what is happening—particularly
in relation to the elements. For example, a good pilot flies a perfectly sound airplane into an ice storm because he or she desires
to get home that night. The pilot was in denial of what was really
happening and consequently went beyond the edge to the point of
no return.

In Phoenix Rising Yoga Therapy sessions I have seen clients who,
as soon as they become aware of the edge in a posture, will begin to
become self-critical, unaccepting or unwilling to be with what is:
"Why can't I go further?" "I'm so inflexible," or "I'm really not suited
to this—it doesn't work for me." It is only by accepting what is happening, no matter what it is, that you can then choose where to go
from there and how to be with it. Then, you can truly play the edge.
(Playing the edge is about making adjustments or fine tuning how
you are, moment to moment.) This takes us even deeper into the
experience, be it a yoga posture or a life experience.

You tend to hold two kinds of tension in your body. First, there is
natural tension. This you need. Without it you would fall over. Then,
there is what is called fear-based tension. This is the kind of tension
you purposely create to keep you safe—out of harm's way. You begin
to do this at an early age. Sometimes you give it up as soon as the
danger is gone and sometimes you keep it. For example, if you are
about to cross a busy road and a car passes close to the sidewalk
before you step off, your body will stiffen a little. After you have

safely crossed the road it will relax. If, however, it was a particularly frightening moment, you may find that every time you go to cross a road from that day on, your body will tighten in fear.

A small child, who I will call Emma, is from an abusive family and she has learned how to use her body to hide. Her shoulders lean forward, her head tilts slightly toward her chest, her eyes are cast towards the floor, and her solar plexus is drawn slightly inward. This posture creates less than a full presence and so, she believes, makes her less visible and lessens the possibility of her being noticed and possibly punished. It works for her. It helps to keep her a little safer. Thirty years later though, when she no longer needs to do this, her body is still doing it. She sometimes doesn't realize she is doing it. It has become a learned strategy and not easy to give up. Her body is still holding this fear-based tension. The first time Emma enters a yoga posture that opens her chest, she meets face-to-face with this old fear. At first it is frightening. If guided to find an edge, she may be able to be present to it. In fact, she may be able to explore it to the extent that it becomes a source of liberation for her. As the feelings and memories are released as the edge moves deeper, her body learns a new way of being; a way of being without the fear-based tension. Surprisingly, she discovers she can let it go and still be safe. The edge has served her well.

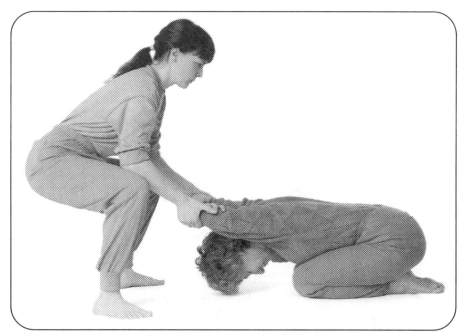

Phoenix Rising Yoga therapist Nancy Nowak helps colleague Stefi Shapiro "let go and be supported."

Exercise

FINDING YOUR EDGE

Drop your head down to the left side bringing your ear toward your shoulder. Notice the stretch this creates on the right side of your neck. Feel the sensation. Breathe into it and let the exhale fall out. Play with the stretch by extending the left arm downward. Imagine you are using the middle two fingers on that hand to reach into a deep pocket for a dime buried deep inside it. Find an edge in the stretch. The edge is the place where any more stretch would be too much, and any less would be not enough. When you find the edge, hang out there for two or three more breaths. Just be with the edge. Notice if it shifts and go with it if it does. Come out of the stretch with your eyes closed and take your inner awareness to both sides of your neck. Check in with yourself physically. Check in with your total awareness of yourself in the moment. What do you find?

Try finding the edge in other body positions. A good one is to explore the edge in the hamstrings by hanging forward like a rag doll with your head hanging down toward your knees. Bend your knees and then slowly begin to straighten them until you find an edge. Use many breaths for this one. As you get better at finding your edge, take it to your yoga practice and then, after a time, see how it translates into your life. How do you tend to play the edge? Do you prefer to push forward or to hang back? How does that serve you? What does it keep you from discovering? How do you choose to be with the edges in your life from here on?

6
Surrender

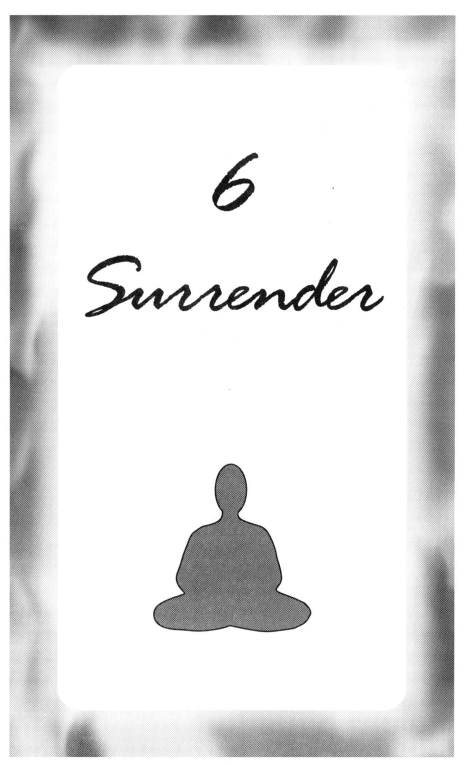

$\mathcal{T}$he word "surrender" conjures up images of defeat for those old enough to remember World War II. It is not something anyone would want to do. It may be seen as a dangerous path: giving up one's freedom, giving up one's mind to the control of another, being weak. To others, especially the yogi in a spiritual sense, surrender implies giving up in some way, and it is one of the most important steps on the path. To surrender is to let go of the "ego-mind." The assumption is that our mind, no matter how great it is and how wonderfully it can rationalize and help us understand our world around us, can never really know it all. The mind might struggle to understand but never really know the mysteries of creation, the very mystery of life itself, the unknowns of the universe. Least of all, the mind is not able to provide us with the one thing we all seek (whether we know we are seeking it or not) and that is an experience of our own Divinity. To the yogi, to experience our Divinity, we must first surrender our "ego-mind."

After a short time as a resident at Kripalu, and having attended some programs there, I saw an opportunity to join the teaching staff. I had been involved in various forms of teaching all of my adult life and had become quite skilled as an instructor. I made my desires known and was quite surprised when told that I needed to wait awhile. Here I was, a "teacher." They really needed teachers and I was making myself available. Instead, I was assigned to a maintenance crew and then later to programs where I was an assistant. At first I thought assisting would be wonderful. At least I would be getting closer to my goal of being on the teaching staff. It turned out to be worse than being on the maintenance crew—much worse. As an assistant, I was reminded every day of my skills as a teacher while not being "allowed" to use them. I was in an inner state of torment. This feeling persisted for some time despite several "processing" sessions with my mentors and senior residents.

Gradually, I began to see what I was doing. My mind was defining me as a teacher and making the perfectly reasonable rationalization that I should be in that role, given my relative skills. On the other hand, I was living in an ashram because I was in search of my soul. Satisfying my mind would, on the surface, make me happier and more comfortable with life. Letting go of it was not easy. But I also had to consider that there may be something wonderful awaiting me on the other side if I could let go. My mind tried to come up with some good reasons for letting go of itself. This proved a very tricky process. Luckily, I had something else going for me—the spiritual lifestyle and the morning yoga and meditation practice. Each morning, I found I could go beyond the struggle with my mind. In those moments, it mattered not whether I was a teacher, a yogi, a janitor or a pilot. In those moments, I was beyond the limiting definition of a role. In those moments I was Divine.

Each day I began to feel the effects of my morning practice lasting longer into the day. I was free from the torment of my perceived limited role for most of the morning. One day I noticed myself actually enjoying the simplicity of my assisting role, handing out paper and pencils. After a few more weeks, I was aware that I had indeed let go. I was no longer in torment. I was enjoying almost every act of the day. The teachers I was working with sought my feedback on their work and I offered it because I genuinely wanted to support them rather than show them how much I knew. Soon, I was also in a teaching role and it was not anywhere near as big a deal as it may have been before. It was just another role. I had moved beyond defining myself in relation to any role—even the one that had defined my identity.

There was also a change in my teaching. I experienced so much more freedom in that role. My whole being was now present to those I taught whereas in the past only the "teacher" part of me could show up. My work was so much more effective and powerful. What a lesson! I now had some understanding of what it meant to surrender. Over the next several years I had many more opportunities to prac-tice this—and it required practice. Of all the lessons I have learned on my journey, I feel that no matter how many times I do it, surren-dering is always an "edge" for me. At the same time, each time I have done it I have been abundantly blessed.

I must add a word of caution here as well. While I believe that learning to surrender was an important step in my spiritual evolu-tion, I also needed to know when not to surrender. I believe there is a need to discriminate between surrendering for the sake of learning to surrender and surrendering as an end-product of manipulation. Unfortunately, it's often difficult to make the distinction—especially from the mind. This is the time to learn how to trust your gut and go with it. More about that later.

Strangely though, as soon as I feel like I have mastered surrender in one area of my life, it will soon show up again in another. For about a year after Lori and I became partners, I resisted the idea of having more children. My first two children were teenagers and I remembered the level of commitment it had required to raise them thus far. I decided not to repeat the experience. Lori, on the other hand, had no children and wanted to experience that part of life. I'm sure this is a struggle for many couples and in telling this story I want to let you know first that I don't believe there is a right or wrong answer to this question when it comes up in a relationship. I would, however, recommend the way I went about resolving it. The process is more important than the answer.

As I had learned so well during my ashram life, the way to solve most of life's problems is to take the question to a higher power than my limited "ego mind." So I did. At this time I was in the process of building my Phoenix Rising Yoga Therapy practice. I was giving a lot in my sessions, which was great, but I knew that I also needed to receive. At this point there were not any other trained Phoenix Rising Yoga therapists, so I sought out an old colleague who practiced a form of deep-tissue bodywork and asked him to work with me. At one point during the session he dug deep into my shoulder blades and found an "edge." I asked him to stay at that place while I breathed and focused my awareness. I sensed he had hit just the right spot. Tears streamed from my closed eyes and I felt a softness in my belly. I felt like a little baby. I began to dialogue with myself to explore it further, asking my friend to stay with the pressure of his thumb under my shoulder blade.

"So little baby what's happening now?"

"I'm fine. I'm having a great time. What's wrong with you?"

"What's wrong with me? Are you kidding?"

"No. I'm just a little baby. I don't kid. I just be me."

"Aaaghh. Damn that hurts! (At this point I notice the part of me that wants to stop the process and just ask my friend to release his pressure and move to another spot. I stay with it.)

"Tell me more."

"I'm the one who is afraid. Afraid of a little baby."

"You big man—afraid of me—a little baby?"

"You got it. I'm afraid of what you'll take from me. My time, my life energy, my freedom to travel, my wife's attention."

"I don't want those things from you."

"You don't?"

"Nah. I just want to be loved."

"But that's what I mean. That takes effort. Time. Presence."

"Hey man, I don't want to be loved that way. I want you to have fun too."

"You do?"

"Sure. What kind of a father would you be if you were miserable about needing to give love? I'll find love whether you give it to me or not. Who says you are the only one who can do that?"

"Okay. I got it. Can we stop this now?"

"You're the boss."

"Geez, what a kid!"

In fact we had to stop at that point as my friend was unable to maintain the pressure, having become incapacitated by laughter. He was hollering and whooping around the room having a great time over my strange conversation with my "child."

I went home and talked with Lori about what had happened. We sat and cried together as she told me that she, too, wanted me to have what I wanted in life, just like the little baby. I told her I wanted the same for her. Together we embraced the possibility of both of us having what we wanted and that it need not take anything from either of us.

A Divine gift came in the form of a son named Joshua. After his birth as I held one hand on his head and one under his buttocks, I had a feeling he was communicating with me. He was asking me for my blessing and for my permission for him to be with me. I gave him a very clear "Yes, my son, yes!" His brother Jack was born three years later and did not need to prepare his path so well. By then I knew the blessings far outweighed the burden. I had surrendered to parenthood.

But I still sometimes struggle with being what I call "the perpetual parent"—now 25 years of it without a break! At other times I feel very blessed. I have a recent memory of Jack learning to swim. It was such a delight to see the grin on his face when he realized he was actually swimming. I will never forget that moment. And when I go to a kindergarten parent/teacher night, for what feels like the hundredth time, I feel like grandpa among the young parents, some barely out of their 20s and me pushing 50. It's a great chance to once again shake loose the concepts that I'm using to create my reality. Lori told me once that in her Middle Eastern culture, each child that is born is seen as the bearer of gifts. At first I laughed about it and didn't buy it. Now I'm beginning to see how it works. I see the gifts, the joy, and the pain, and surrender to all.

By Divine coincidence, about the time of Joshua's birth I was working with a client named Ellie who desperately tried for several years to have children. Both Ellie and her husband had infertility examinations which came up negative but after several more months of trying there was still no baby. During one session after a considerable physical release around her shoulders during an assisted chest-opening posture, she sat in a crossed-leg position as I guided her in meditation. She took her time to speak after the meditation and I could see from her expression that something had affected her deeply. She told me that during the meditation she received guidance. She had learned that her desire to have children came from her desire to love. She also learned that whether she had children of her own or not, it would not affect her capacity to love and that what she really wanted to create in her life was an opportunity to love. Sometime later she told me that they had made arrangements to adopt a baby from Korea. By the time she and her husband were scheduled to receive their daughter, she was pregnant.

Now, they have two daughters six months apart from different parts of the world. Ellie's story is yet again confirmation to me of the power of appropriate surrender. She was able to get all she had ever wanted. I believe her willingness to let go of wanting life to give it to her in a particular form was the key to her receiving such a blessing.

Ed's story was similar. In the first few sessions, Ed had made quite a lot of noise in his release in various postures and there had been no connection to any event or circumstance in his life. In his third session, he began to cry and during the integration at the end of the session he reported feeling angry with his father and his grandfather. His anger came from the awareness that neither of these powerful men would accept him until he passed their test. The test was that he do something "outstanding" with his life. From what he could gather, both of these men held the view that if one did not do something "outstanding" with their life then they did not deserve to be alive. Ed was 42 years old and as yet had done nothing "outstanding" enough to satisfy his elders. Ed had done some pretty wonderful things, including establishing a successful *shiatsu* practice and gaining respect in the local community. To Ed though, this did not count. He was just biding his time. Sooner or later, he felt, he would have to reenter the corporate world he had left a few years earlier and prove himself a man. He frowned a lot and told me when we began to work that he longed for a lasting and loving relationship in his life. He now saw how he could never have such a relationship as long as he had not accomplished something "outstanding." Until that time, he was less than a complete man, according to his father and grandfather. He allowed himself to feel the anger and to take in the new awareness that he had been mislead. That hurt. After all, he loved these men dearly and they had been strong influences in his life.

The awareness had come to him in the assisted posture we had been doing that day. For a time, while in the posture and when he came out of it, he felt the presence of a Higher Power. That Higher Power was his own spirit. It told him that he was perfect just the way he was. There was nothing he needed to do to prove himself to anyone. All he needed was within him. His only task was to listen to his truth and follow its guidance. This was so difficult for him, even though he knew it was what he needed and wanted to do. His grandfather was in his late 90s. He didn't want to displease him before his death. He desperately wanted to reconnect with his father who had partly rejected him since Ed had resigned his corporate position. Ed didn't know what to do. He wanted to surrender to his Higher Power but didn't know how. I asked him if he would like to go back into the posture again and give it a try. He said he would like that, so we did. He emerged saying he felt more courageous and willing to let go. He had handed over to his Higher Power the responsibility for his father and grandfather. He was going to continue to love them both and continue to follow his inner guidance rather than try to win their approval by meeting their expectations. I wished him well and didn't see him again for some time.

One day he came into my office without the frown. He came to invite me to his wedding and to let me know that he had made peace with his father by sharing with him his commitment to follow his inner guidance. His father understood in essence what he was saying and although he had struggled with the direction that he seemed to be taking, he acknowledged that Ed had to live his own life. He apologized for forcing his expectations upon him. He had been in therapy himself recently and could see how he had projected his own fears onto Ed. Ed was totally amazed by this outcome. His act of surrender had given him all he had ever wanted from his father.

It is difficult for my conscious mind to do this act of surrender without help. To let go I need to be free of mind-generated fears and restrictions. The best way I know of doing this is to use my body as the means of being present to myself. It's amazing how soft I can get with myself after just two or three minutes in a supported yoga posture taking deep, releasing breaths.

Exercise

OPENING UP TO SURRENDER IN YOUR LIFE

Sit on your heels on the floor. Use pillows under your buttocks or ankles if you need to. Place another pillow on the floor in front of you. Join your hands behind your back and come forward slowly from the waist, placing your head on the pillow in front of you. (Be careful not to hyper-extend the back of your neck. The cervical spine should be perpendicular to the floor and the weight on the crown of your head). Raise both arms up behind your back until you find an edge. Focus awareness into the sensations and breathe deep, falling-out breaths. You are now in a variation of the Yoga *Mudra*—a posture that symbolically is about the essence of yoga. It is the posture of surrender. It is about the surrender of the ego-mind to allow the opening to the soul—the Higher Self. As you hold the posture allow yourself to let go in all other aspects of your being. Ask to surrender all that keeps you separate from your soul. This might include fears, habits, old beliefs that no longer serve you or anything in the way of your continued transformation. Come slowly out of the posture and sit quietly in meditation. Ask your Higher Self for guidance. When you receive it write it down.

7

Teachers
and Gurus

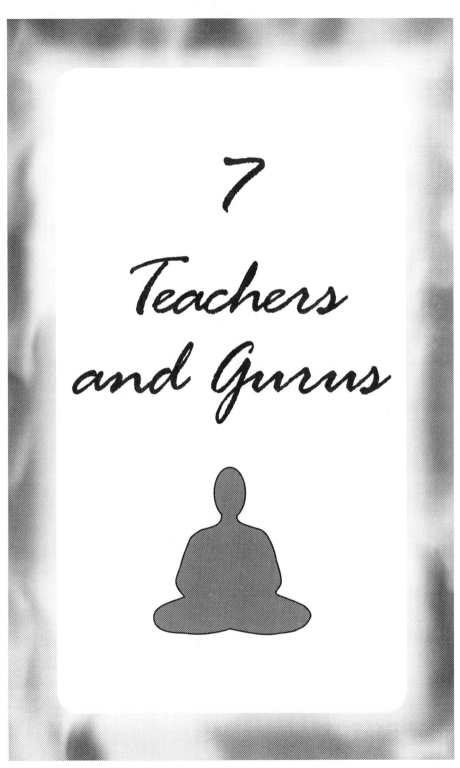

*T*o some extent, yoga and gurus seem to go together like bread and butter. But is a guru really an essential part of the package for us as we follow the yogic path in life? Is a teacher essential, or can we find own own path?

Traditionally in yoga, the guru/disciple relationship is based on the idea that for a person to progress spiritually it is necessary to surrender the "ego mind," as discussed earlier. The teacher or guru serves this purpose. Assuming the teacher knows more about the spiritual path and is enlightened enough to teach the student how to progress spiritually, then it stands to reason that the teacher will help the student move more quickly along the path to spiritual wisdom. Along the way, however, the student will confront resistance, particularly if the ego is strong. In our youth, if our self-concept is reasonably healthy, we will get to a place in life where we really believe we have it figured out. We think we have all of the answers and often don't realize that there is much that we truly don't know. We usually need to encounter some moments in which we surrender to not knowing so as to be able to learn what we don't yet know.

On the other hand, one of the advantages of youthful exuberance is that we position ourselves in life with great regularity to set up experiences that will teach us. Often such experiences are not pleasant but we learn. They may include experimentation with alcohol or drugs, venturing into unknown neighborhoods, frequenting previously off-limits places and so on. I recall, as a youth, the experience of being ill from overindulging in alcohol. I repeated the experience maybe a handful of times before I learned that it was something I would prefer to avoid. I quickly learned that a more moderate approach to drinking was my path of preference. Would I, or could I, have learned this more easily if some chosen teacher had verbally enlightened me before the event and prevented me from the uncomfortable experiences? Maybe, maybe not. Sometimes we have to hack around on our own before we are ready to accept coaching. Experience can be a great teacher by itself and in many cases, mastery is achieved in a field just through trial and error. Pioneers in aviation had no coaches or instructors. They were the first. The results of some of their early experiences were not very successful and at times they were fatal. But others learned from their experiences and they flew.

Often, experience itself will point the way toward finding a teacher or at least collaborating with others to find a better way. I'm sure those early aviators were eager to learn from each other whenever possible. How many golfers learn the game by themselves, only to find later as they improve a little, that they might do better with some serious coaching?

One of the problems with having a teacher is of course the requirement to surrender to some extent, regardless of whether we are learning golf, learning how to fly an airplane or learning the game of life through yoga.

In the Zen tradition it is said we need to empty our mind and unlearn all that we already know. It's a risky thing to do. What if we really *do* know and the teacher pretends to know but really doesn't? What if the teacher knows a lot but doesn't know how to teach it? Or how about the methods? All coaches use their own approach to coaching. Some are kind and understanding, some are brutal. How do we know which method will work for us? There is also the question of the teacher's personal life. Would it work to have a golf coach who drank too much and abused her children? Must a spiritual teacher be spiritually pure and practice what he teaches in order to be helpful to others on the spiritual path? Must a flight instructor be an ace pilot herself or just know how to fly and know how to teach it? Could we surrender in good faith to such questionable coaches or teachers? Or doesn't it matter? Is it not the result that *really* matters? If I have a coach or learn on my own, or if I have a pure coach or a questionable coach, may really not be the issue. What *really* matters is whether or not I attain my goal, and whether or not the processes I am choosing to do so, are working for me or not. Am I giving myself the best possible chance of getting to where I want to go by using the methods I've chosen?

Such a question however, shifts the responsibility for success from coach to student. Many of us do not like such a situation. We would prefer to have someone else take that responsibility. Such a question also implies that we engage in a process of self-monitoring and process evaluation as we go along and be prepared to change tracks at any time if we find we are not getting to where we want to go, or if something doesn't seem right with the process. We need to be an empowered, questioning, self-monitoring student, not a passive, unthinking, out-of-touch recipient of what is being taught. You may think the former state of being is incompatible with the idea of surrender, but I think not. Surrender doesn't mean sacrifice. I don't have to give up my own feel for life to surrender to someone's coaching. I can surrender and be vigilant at the same time.

When I arrived at the Kripalu Center in early 1984, I believed I had found my spiritual home. I was attracted to the tranquility, serenity and the loving open-heartedness that came from most of the residents. I had heard a lot about "Gurudev"—as Yogi Desai was known. I thought he must be a very special human being because of the deep devotion and respect that the residents lavished upon him. I was disappointed in my first encounter with him as we passed on a stairwell. He seemed to me just like an ordinary human being. As I spent more time in his presence, I had a better understanding of what it was that made him so attractive to his disciples. He exuded an energy in his presence and in his speaking, that touched me deeply. He was able to directly address spiritual questions that I had never articulated and that seemed to reside deep within my own knowing. In his presence the inadequacies I felt as a loving and deeply spiritual human being were often dissolved. Sometimes after just 20 minutes in meditation, I began to feel like a living saint. I experienced a serene sense of inner peace, I was in love with the world, with life and with myself. It was great. There was nowhere else I wanted to be. I was home. Like most of my colleagues, I attributed my good fortune in this aspect of self-discovery, to being in the presence of a living master— someone able to light my spiritual fire through his mere presence. What I did not appreciate then, was that I was the doer and he was the catalyst. I was the fertile ground in which the seeds were sown and he was merely providing the fertilizer.

In May 1984, I was initiated as a disciple of Amrit Desai. It was not an easy decision for me to make. At first I resisted it, thinking that I would have to behave like many of the *bhakti* (devotional) disciples whose outward showing of devotion to the guru left me puzzled. The devotional path was not for me. Being an Australian of Irish descent with a long family history of contempt for rulers and royalty, I could not bring myself to indulge in great acts of reverence for any fellow human being. I was also afraid of selling myself out. If I became a disciple and surrendered to the guru, would this be the end of my individuality and autonomy? This was a dilemma I discussed with some of the long-term residents. One friend asked me what my experience had been like since I had arrived at the ashram. I told him it had been wonderful. He said to just trust my experience, and that, in itself would help me make my decision. I took that as sound advice. During the pre-initiation retreat I also discovered that the aspect of surrender in the guru/disciple relationship was a surrender to our inner guru (our own internal Higher Power) and that the external guru merely reflected the inner guru to the seeker. This knowledge, together with my wonderful experience living there, was enough to convince me.

I felt I could make use of the guru/disciple relationship to learn and at the same time I continued to monitor the process to ensure it was serving me. I was prepared to surrender to learn and yet at the same time was watchful of the implications each time I had to make the choice to surrender. It was an interesting time. I was also aware of how many of my guru brothers and sisters took surrender to extremes that were beyond my understanding. At times I had self-doubt when I saw this. The extent to which some of my colleagues compromised their lifestyle for the sake of surrender was further than I could ever take it. I remember thinking that maybe I was missing something because I couldn't see myself in their place and maybe I hadn't been around long enough to learn what surrender really was. Not long after, I experienced a situation that gave me the opportunity to distinguish between trusting in my own knowing and surrendering to authority in a situation where there were motives beyond those pertaining to my spiritual advancement.

I was co-leading a program with a senior colleague who one morning announced that he would be teaching the session that day instead of me. He said that he needed to do it to "lift" the program. I felt angry, humiliated and bewildered. My own inner knowing was that I was doing a great job. It didn't make sense but there was no time to argue and he was the senior teacher so I acquiesced.

Later with no clarity around the issue and still feeling confused by his decision, I slowly began to distance myself from him. I found it hard to trust my inner knowing and to trust him. Although I was being called to surrender, there was something that didn't feel right to me. I was also sad as my relationship with this person had been very close. The wound went deep. I had to surrender to what was happening and also deal with my inner truth. Not teaching the session was the easy part. I could let go of that. What I could not let go of was my inner knowing that something did not ring true. His explanation did not make any sense to me as only the day before he had praised my work highly. A voice inside said "trust yourself and what you know to be true," yet that was difficult.

If I hadn't been able to find that trust in myself, I would have found it very difficult to ever walk in front of another group in a teaching role. Although I couldn't fully understand it, my way of dealing with it was to make an inner prayer and commitment. It went like this:

> God, I know I am not perfect and I have much to learn. I also know that I am loved. I am open to learning what I need to learn. At the same time I will not allow my doubts, my fears, and my imperfections to keep me from being present to what I know in my heart to be true. Please help me.

It worked. I began to shake the self-doubt that was disempowering me and to believe again that I was more than enough for my teaching role.

This experience also served me greatly in the years ahead. As all teachers know, there are times when you will trigger feelings in your students. Often these feelings will be projected onto you as the teacher. With experience as a teacher you learn to look at what is coming at you and make a choice whether it's something you need to look at seriously for your own growth or whether it's something being projected at you that you can give back to the student. It's a hard call and sometimes you get it right and sometimes you don't. Each time you don't, you learn something and have a better chance next time at getting it, as long as you don't go under. Teachers who learn to do this well, generally are able to take greater risks and become more powerful and effective teachers. I am grateful for the circumstances in 1984 that pushed me to the edge with that process. They helped me find a deeper level of trust in myself. For many years though, I was saddened by my loss of faith and trust in my colleague and the loss of his friendship.

Ten years later, the same colleague was a dinner guest in my home. Prior to that visit, we had had several interactions with each other over the years and at times even acknowledged the bond that had existed between us but was no more. At the same time, there was still the awful feeling of something not being quite right in our relationship. In the spring of 1994, we had connected again at a conference. In one of many conversations, my friend shared his desire to talk to me and tell me the truth about what had happened. He, along with many long-term Kripalu residents were finding it increasingly difficult to continue the guru/disciple relationship with Yogi Desai. He spoke of how he had sold himself out to the guru and expressed his deep hurt and anger about that. At dinner he told me about what had happened 10 years earlier. It seems that one of the participants in the program that we'd taught together in 1984, was a generous financial supporter of the ashram. She had made a strong connection with him as a student of one of his previous programs and was disappointed that he was not the sole teacher of the current program so she could strengthen her connection to him. She had complained to one of the senior administrators who, in turn, instructed my colleague to pull me out to satisfy the donor and keep her financial support. He did so but was in a dilemma. He didn't feel he could tell me the truth without being disloyal to her and thus indirectly to the guru. At the same time he knew the hurt it caused me and the rift it created in our relationship. He was now apologizing and asking for my forgiveness, 10 years later. Given how the situation had served to empower me, I forgave him easily and felt great compassion for him. He asked me to express my hurt and my disappointment to help him feel the impact of his actions. His deep desire to clean up a major issue in his life impressed me. He, and other residents had begun to realize they had been selling themselves out in the name of the guru/disciple relationship. They had taken their surrender to extremes that compromised their inner integrity.

The subsequent developments and discoveries around this issue over the following years resulted in major changes at Kripalu and a complete turn away from the guru/disciple relationship as the foundation of spiritual practice there. This, however, is a subject worthy of another book and too massive to detail here.

Fortunately for me, I was able to distinguish when it was appropriate to surrender and when to take a stand, even though sometimes I was initially confused.

Lori and I began dating in 1986. We were not supposed to be dating. She was a resident of the ashram and although by then, I was living in a nearby community, I was an ex-resident, teacher, and community member and I was supposed to continue to follow the ashram's guidelines which limits contact between male and female members of the community. We were seen holding hands on a street in a nearby town and asked by one of the directors to explain our action and how it supported our chosen lifestyle. We admitted to our relationship and love for each other. Lori chose to go for an indefinite period to the smaller ashram in Sumneytown, Pennsylvania, to contemplate her intentions. After a brief period there, we both decided we would rather be together than follow the guidance offered to us at that time. Lori moved out and we have been together since. As a result of our choice we were "banned" from going to the ashram for six months on the basis that our decision would affect others and we should not be seen there in a relationship. This was painful for both of us. It was our spiritual home and almost all our friends lived there. But we felt clear in our decision and waited out the time and then reconnected again. How pleased I am today that we chose that course. As difficult as it was, we had allowed our own inner truth to take precedence over the choice to simply surrender to the organization's guidelines.

I have no regrets that I took that action. My time at the ashram had served me well. I grew spiritually in three significant ways. First, I opened my heart. Inspired by the teachings, I found the love inside of me that enabled me to wash away many of my old fears and find greater peace and serenity in my life. Second, I learned to get my ego out of my way enough to be present without the need to wear the mask of a role identity. In doing this, I could be present to myself and others in ways that I could not have imagined. Third, I learned to deepen my trust in myself and to go against the grain to make difficult choices and honor my inner truth. I no longer need a guru. Yet spending time around a teacher who could help me reach deep into my spirit, served me well. I was fortunate in that I had a relatively healthy relationship with both of my parents. I had no difficulty speaking with them and I am grateful for their love and support. Given this, I was clearly not seeking a guru to substitute for unfulfilled parental love. I was also not seeking the answer to my salvation. If anything, I was looking to be part of a family that seemed like it was doing something wonderful in the world in a loving way. I knew I could learn a lot by being a part of it. And I did. Rarely was I tempted to see the guru as superhuman, although I can understand how easy it was for some to see him that way. To me he was always a man—like me. And like me, he had some very special skills and knowledge and could use them to support me and others in our transformational process in a profound way. He also had a dark side just like me, which could influence his decisions and judgment as easily as his open-hearted spirit could. And when his judgment erred he would someday have to account for it and learn from it, either in this lifetime or the hereafter—just like me or any human being—perfectly imperfect.

When it came down to choices significantly affecting my life, I could listen and take note of the guru's teachings and guidance but I had to also listen to my own truth and check it out. I can see how easily surrender can become repression. It's a fine edge and requires much inner vigilance to stay in integrity with one's inner truth. One

must walk the edge between surrender and will, learning to distinguish between the voice of the ego and the voice of the soul. In
ancient India and in many other spiritual cultures, it was often
assumed that the individual was unable to walk such an edge. Total
surrender was encouraged to a teacher who could reflect only the
soul. I am uncertain if such teachers ever really existed then, or do
exist today. Perhaps so. But either way, the ultimate surrender must
be to the enlightened being that lives within us, so why not start
getting in touch with it as soon as possible? As I reflect in hindsight,
I believe many guru/disciple relationships can be useful and very
beneficial or as codependent and dysfunctional as any other relationship. Sooner or later though, I believe that we must kick away
the support structure and stand on our own two spiritual feet, trusting in our own inner wisdom in all matters both spiritual as well as
material.

I also see a very healthy phenomenon emerging in our society as
we enter the 21st century. There is a paradigm shift occurring in
regard to our relationships. The last 100 years of the 20th century
saw a massive upheaval and shifting of power in many previously
accepted hierarchical relationships. Relationships between races and
between sexes have been irreversibly changed. The playing field has
been leveled and that has been a positive move for all. Relationships
are moving toward authenticity rather than assigned power. There
are signs that we are growing up and learning how to relate with a
degree of maturity and authenticity never before experienced. Given
this, I believe the guru/disciple relationship, though clearly useful to
some, is an option and not an essential prerequisite to the spiritual
path of the Western world in the 21st century.

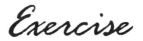

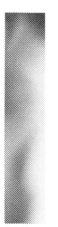

An Introspective Experience

Sit quietly and meditate for a few moments witnessing or counting your breaths. Let your focus be inward. When you feel calm and relaxed, ask yourself, "How much more or less power do I give to others to influence what I do in my life today, compared to what I did 10 years ago? How does this feel?" Check out the feelings in your body as you hold the questions and the answers. What is your body telling you? When you come out of the meditation, journal your thoughts, feelings and awareness.

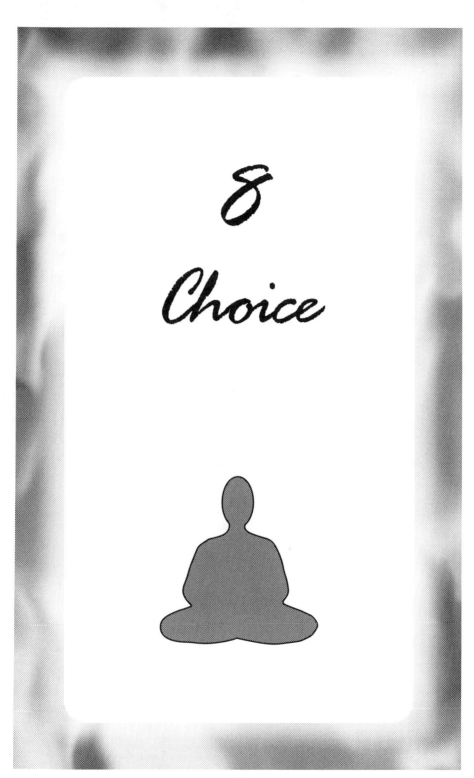

8

Choice

*W*e were conducting a training program in Dallas. Not having spent much time there, I had an image of Dallas as a brash and materialistic city probably without much soul. I was soon to let go of my prejudice. In the elevator of my hotel on my way to the program, I almost doubled over in delight when a young woman dressed in black evening wear hitched her dress up to scratch her thigh exclaiming, "Damn! These new panty-hose are so itchy." She wasn't drunk. Her date standing next to her looked like a Fortune 500 executive and she was just being herself. I was impressed. It was so different from the heavily censored public behavior I observe in New England where I live. Over and over again in Texas I had a chance to witness folks just "being themselves." Now that doesn't mean this freedom of expression was always pretty or filled with consciousness awareness, but it was real. For the first time in many years I tuned in the car radio to a country station and as I listened to the lyrics I noticed a similar realness. Sure, a lot of the songs are about attachment, disappointment and bravado, but again they are real. Even if you don't like the lyrics, I see that the big resurgence in the popularity of this style of music is due to a certain down-to-earth quality in it. I decided I liked Dallas after all.

When I went home and told Lori I liked Dallas, she responded, "Great! But don't you realize you like every city you visit?" She was right. Although I wouldn't like to live in all of them, I do seem to find something I like about each of them. I think the way I am with cities is also a great way to be with people. We can either focus on what it is about someone that drives us crazy or we can focus on something about them we like. Just as you do with a city, you have to be with someone long enough to be able to do that. Time and time again, in training programs and workshops, I see people connecting deeply with so many people they have spent time with, who are different from themselves.

I have often asked how this is so? How can people taking a Phoenix Rising training program suddenly become able to accept major differences in others that they find difficulty with elsewhere? Are they mesmerized by the program? Is it an "unreal" situation? I think not. What I think happens is that after even just a short time in the program people shift gears. From this new state of being they begin to see more than their initial prejudice. How does this happen? I think it's a combination of things. First, we place a lot of emphasis on the use of the body as a vehicle for deeper awareness. On the first morning, within a half hour of arriving, people are led through their first body experience. We guide them through a series of partner yoga postures and at the same time use the physical experience as a way of focusing awareness inward. It's done in a way that is not too threatening and not very physically challenging. It's also a lot of fun. By the time the exercise is over, people have become introspective at a fairly deep level. We also work on using physical acceptance as a key to whole-person self-acceptance. Once I begin to more fully accept myself, I begin to more fully accept others. Whatever I am afraid to acknowledge in myself, I most certainly don't like to see in others. If there is a lot that I don't accept in myself, there is a lot in others that troubles me. My choices of who I can relate to become much more limited. What I don't like in the other, becomes a barrier to being with them long enough to discover what I appreciate. I have closed the window before I have even taken a good look through it. What I see happening as people become more aware and more self-accepting through their bodies is that they open up more choices for themselves in relationship to others.

I also believe that our insecurity in our beliefs limits our choices. When I first became a vegetarian, I found reasons to dislike people who ate meat. Somehow I wanted to make them wrong in order to make myself right. Why did I need to make myself right? Because at a deep, honest-to-goodness, soul-searching level, I wasn't totally convinced that being vegetarian was right for me. I needed to make it right. I needed to support my new behavior with a firm and true conviction. Of course, on the surface, I appeared totally clear about my decision. Deep down though, there was doubt that I was unwilling to acknowledge. Some years later, when I widened my diet to include occasional seafood and dairy products, I became accepting of what others chose to eat and did not label them according to their dietetic choices. I had found a way of being with myself that worked for me and so I assumed that others could do the same for themselves. Since external behavior matched my internal beliefs, there was no longer a need for others to act in a certain way to make me feel better about my beliefs.

In Phoenix Rising we use body-oriented processes to help us get in touch with our deep inner beliefs. They are often not what we think they are. They are often more universal and accommodating of our humanity than they are dogmatic. For example, when I am focused inwardly through my body and I am totally present to myself, and I ask myself about diet, I get a response like this, "What you choose to eat is important because you need to take care of your body in the best way you can." At the same time, your body will also help you and take care of you. It is a partnership. Like a good partner, your body is also very forgiving when it needs to be. "You must be gentle with yourself. Choose things that are good for you but don't create resistance by being too dogmatic about it. If you trust yourself to make good choices moment-to-moment it will serve you better than having a rigid formula to live by." When I am out of touch, not focused inwardly and following only my mind, what I get is, "You must be a total vegetarian—it is the only way." I know which counsel I prefer. I also know that when I am guided in my beliefs and my behavior by my inner wisdom, I am much more open to the differences in others. I know that they, if they are in touch with their truth, will get the guidance that is right for them. It may or may not be similar to mine and it doesn't really matter. If they are not in touch with their truth and they are living from a dogmatic mind, so be it. Eventually it may serve them to look deeper when they realize that their dogmatism doesn't serve them anymore.

So when we take the time to be fully present to ourselves it's so much easier to be fully present to others. In being fully present, the masks drop away. Under the masks, if we go deep enough, there is a delightful human spirit with which we can connect. What helps us get to that place? One of the ways is to consciously choose what we emphasize when connecting with the other. Often we don't see it as a choice. We just see the ugliness and never the beauty and relate from that place. To have a choice we have to be willing to take the time to look a little further—to be present enough to see more, feel more, experience more than just what comes to us on the surface.

Beth was petite and soft-spoken. On the third day of the Level One training program, after a partner exchange, she rejoined the group and shared her experience. While she was holding a particular posture we were practicing, she said she had a flash of awareness about how she creates pain in her life as a way of avoiding being powerful. She had noticed the discomfort and how, despite the discomfort, she could change her experience moment-to-moment. She could use her concentration to turn it into pain or into something joyfully pleasant. She noticed herself repeatedly choosing pain. She noticed how choosing pain made her feel weak. She noticed the moments when she chose joy instead of pain and how that choice made her feel strong. It was difficult for her to choose joy, because pain was a more familiar and comfortable feeling for her. On the other hand, the glimpse she got of her power felt good, too, albeit scary. She wasn't sure what to do with this new awareness. I asked her to notice when it came up in her life and to allow herself to be any way she might want to be with it, but to be aware of the choices she had rather than just acting on "auto pilot." Little did we know at the time that she would have a great opportunity to do this within the next few hours.

The next morning she was late. We knew she had to take her daughter to day-care and we assumed that she was delayed in traffic. She arrived after about 15 minutes and I noticed a delightful smile on her face as she settled in. As we were finishing up our morning check-in, she asked if she could tell us what had happened to her. It seems that the previous evening as she approached her house, she noticed a car accident right in front of it. To her surprise, one of the cars belonged to her husband. On his way to collect their daughter, he had "spaced-out" coming out of the driveway and had hit an oncoming car. No one was injured but the cars were badly damaged. Once she knew that he was okay she went on to pick up their daughter while her husband rested. On her way home she began noticing the pain she felt about the accident. For months she had been asking her husband not to work so hard. He worked all day with computers and then worked several more hours glued to the computer screen at home. She observed how his life had become imbalanced and wanted him to put it in harmony. She realized how easy it would be for her to go home and say, "See? I told you so! You work so much that you 'spaced-out' and look what happened." But through the pain she felt grateful that he hadn't been hurt. She was grateful for his willingness to pick up the children and to support her in her decision to take the training program. She began to see that she had a clear choice. She could return home carrying either pain or gratitude. She chose the latter.

As she walked in the door she saw from both his body posture and facial expression, that her husband expected to get her disapproval and her pain. Instead, she put her arms around him and said, "I'm so pleased you were not hurt." He then told her how awful he felt about it, how he needed to change his ways and be more focused, and a whole lot more. She listened with love, just as she had been learning to do in her training, and gave him room to feel his feelings and to be received by her just as he was. Out of the drama of a car accident came some of the most loving moments that each of them had experienced for some time. If that was the only result of her new-found capacity to choose, it would have been enough, but there was more.

Later in the program, Beth told us that she and her husband were now exploring many facets of their lives and their relationship together. They were planning to share more family time together and other ways of bringing their lives more into balance with their intentions. The conversations she had often longed for were now happening. As well as being wonderful, it was also scary. She was discovering a whole lot more about her husband, and he about her. There was a danger that as they got to know each other more, they may not like what they found. To Beth, though, it was a risk worth taking. She had now been emotionally free of pain for several days and she loved it. Not surprisingly, she also noticed she was free of physical pain in her right shoulder which had been with her for years.

Beth's story clearly illustrates how our willingness to be present to ourselves enhances our capacity to be present to others. Beth's willingness to be present to herself and her awareness of her pain opened the door for her to move beyond it. Once she did, the whole universe around her began to change as she made new choices.

Another area of choice that is worth exploring is how you choose to do the things you have to do anyway—often those onerous little tasks that are essential to your life but may not be all that important in any given moment. I remember as a small boy, hearing my father's reprimand, "If something is not worth doing well then it's not worth doing at all!" I remember thinking, "But, Dad, there are so many things to do and they are all so exciting, I can't possibly get to do them all if I have to do them all well." It was probably fear that he wouldn't understand that kept me from voicing these words and they remained my secret "knowing." I learned to adapt—doing well the things that might come under his careful scrutiny, and doing other things just well enough to get the job done so I could be free to move on. It was only after some years that I began to question this particular life strategy.

I remember washing dishes one day with my friend Brendan. Brendan has the wonderful quality of being able to enjoy life in most situations. We had just finished sharing dinner with friends who had to leave as soon as the meal was completed and there we were with a mountain of dishes to wash. I began to complain about the amount of time it was going to take us to complete the task. Brendan offered a suggestion. "Why don't we wash each and every plate, pot or fork in a way that it has never been washed before—with absolute excellence?" I surrendered to his idea—after all, we had to do something to entertain ourselves. To my surprise, our "game" began to have an amazing effect. What had been an onerous chore became a joy. I found myself getting mildly excited as I picked up the next plate and greeted it with the sponge. Washing each plate was a new, unique and fulfilling experience. I chose to be totally present to each dish for each moment I washed it. The time passed quickly and the gleaming plates seemed to smile at us reflecting my "inner smile" as we finished. I remembered that event and applied what I'd learned from it to many future situations.

The dishwashing experience later connected with one of my early experiences in a yoga community. It was at Ananda Ashram in the Sierra Nevadas of California in the late 1970s. There hung a sign over the door of the little cabin that served as the guest registration office, that read, "The Guest Is God." I began to observe, during my stay there, how the resident community really worked to give meaning to those words. By choosing to serve us in this way, the Divine nature of each of us began to emerge. There was a quality in the way people related to each other resulting from the chosen intention of seeing God in each other. I remember thinking, "Just like washing dishes—it works with people too!"

A similar experience occurred when I first came to Kripalu. My first job was with the maintenance crew and my task was to replace the knobs on many doors. After the first few days I began to become very casual in my approach to the task. Even the gentle reminder from one of my colleagues didn't inspire me at first. Then I remembered the dishes. Ahh! Now I would do doorknobs with excellence. That lasted a few more days after which the "enjoyment" or "ego gratification," as I was to soon learn, had worn off. I was back in misery with the task. Then I began to watch my mind. The "dishes" approach had worked for a while but I tried to imagine what it would be like to do each task of putting on a doorknob as a meditation—total focus on each moment without expectation, without effort. I tried it. By the end of the day I felt alive, happy and different. The difference was that I had done a day's work and wasn't at all concerned about what I had achieved. I didn't even need to know I had done an excellent job, or that anyone else knew. There was a kind of emptiness as though I had let go of a part of my old self and it was a little scary. How would I get real gratification if my ego was not in my work? It was a beginning. I tried on this new posture over the next several months. It made a tremendous difference to many things, but in particular to my teaching. I found myself easily being present with each moment as I taught. No longer invested in the outcome or in the praise I would get, I was free to be present with a quality of excellence.

I was recently reminded of all this when I arrived to lead a workshop at Song of the Morning Ranch in northern Michigan. There, on a sign in the driveway, was the name of the place with the subheading "A yoga retreat of excellence." The serene beauty of the location was equally matched by the careful attention to detail, without obsession, given by the staff to the guests. The resulting energy of the place was welcoming and inviting. This made it easy for the participants to be open to themselves and each other during our workshop there. It reminded me of how important it is for us in our Phoenix Rising sessions and in our training programs to pay close attention to the detail that creates excellence. Even more important is the attitude with which we do it. If it's "just another chore," it could seem like the dishes that I saw as I complained. If it's seen as an opportunity to choose a state of being without ego attachment, then it will truly serve the higher purpose of transformation.

Exercise

EXPRESS YOUR APPRECIATION WITH LOVE

PART 1.

Lie face down on the floor, bring your hands up under your shoulders, head to the center, and then slowly let your upper body rise from the floor, putting a little weight into your arms and come up into the cobra posture. Hold the posture and breathe deeply. As you hold the posture consciously choose, moment-to-moment, how you want to be with it. Explore all the different stories, feelings, etc. that you allow your mind to focus on as you hold the posture. Then choose a focus. Hold a few more breaths with that focus and then come down.

PART 2.

Think of a city you have visited. Think about what it is in particular that you like about it. Feel yourself being there and feeling what that is like for you in your body.

That was a warm-up exercise.

Now think of a person who is a key player in your life. Look closely at your relationship and find a way that you habitually relate to this person which doesn't create what you want in the relationship. That is, some way you continually show up for this person out of habit—a way in which you relate out of habit rather than out of *choice*.

One of my favorites is walking in the door of my house, noticing something out of place, and remarking on it before greeting anyone in the house. I have come to see how this choice, or lack thereof, disturbs the energy in my house and closes off the deep connection I'm looking for with my family. So I want to break the habit. Now, before I come through the door, I pause, take a deep breath, open up my chest and get in touch with the love I feel in my heart for my family. I remind myself to greet whoever I meet when I open the door, with all the love I feel for them before doing anything else. In doing this I will be acting in accord with my priorities in life. A neat house may be important to me but not more important than the love I feel for my family, so it can wait. First I must express my love.

When you have discovered an unproductive habit of your own, work it through like my example. Try to find a body posture that helps you to focus inward and to go beyond the habit to a deeper level of intention. You can find this by asking yourself what is *really* important to you in life. Opening my chest with deep breaths always works for me to find a more loving place. If it's a stronger posture you are looking for you might want to lengthen your spine, breathe into your belly and plant your feet firmly on the ground. Whatever you come up with has to be real, so make sure you are affirming something in the relationship that is true for you. Then practice. Next time you are

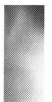

about to come into the presence of the person again, try on the body posture first and then focus into your deeper level of choice. Using the body in this way as an opening to exercising a different choice in behavior can make a significant difference to the quality of any relationship.

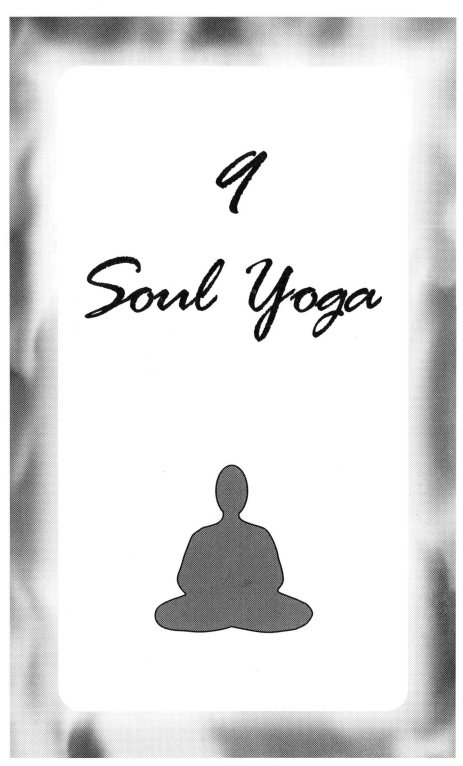

9
Soul Yoga

*T*he amazing material "development" that has occurred in our world in the past century, has been largely linked with the development of our mental capacity as a species. It took great minds to put a human being into orbit around the Earth and then on the moon. To achieve such feats required great analytical ability. In day-to-day life in our modern world we have become good at making distinctions, sorting, separating, categorizing, analyzing and using logic to solve problems. All of these are useful capabilities, if not essential to life in the 20th century. If applied universally, however, such capabilities can also be limiting.

It is interesting to note how different disciplines in the healing arts lay claim to specific parts of our being. A lot of time and energy has gone into drawing up these demarcation boundaries. Psychologists can only work with matters pertaining to the mind, surgeons only with the body, ministers of religion only with healing the human spirit, and so on. Often these demarcations are more about the safeguard of power than about what is best for the individual. Having grown up in Australia, I remember various periods of industrial unrest in the nation as the different trade unions fought with each other for control and power. Such conflicts were referred to as "demarcation disputes." We have much the same situation today in relation to who owns the right to work with our bodies, our minds, our spirits and our overall well-being. For many years, chiropractors fought for a place of legitimacy in the health-care arena and were bitterly opposed by others concerned with the safeguard of power. There are even power struggles occurring in the realm of the holistic healing arts. Various professional associations are vying for the sole right to decide who should, or who should not, be allowed to practice a particular therapy.

I know from experience that there is another side to this. It is important that the general public is able to identify who is trained and who is certified to practice a particular modality. At the same time there must be room for anyone who wishes to enter the arena to be able to do so and to be directly accountable through consumer protection laws to the public they serve. The public should also have access to information on which to base an educated choice of services. In an ideal society, there would be freedom and accountability rather than restriction, control and manipulation to preserve power.

Sometimes it seems as if there is a small pie to be divided with several parties trying to grab the biggest piece. We as human and spiritual beings, are somewhat of a "problem pie." We don't take too well to being divided because somehow all the pieces are connected and have bits of each other contained within. Modern physics tells us that one single cell contains the complete blueprint of who we are. We have grappled for thousands of years with the strange, yet seemingly true, notion that we are at the very same time both nothing and everything. We are the smallest atom and the entire universe at the same time. Our minds have a hard time with that concept but when we go beyond the mind and into experience, there are many of us who have gone far enough into those experiences to know that the concept is actually true in practice. We get glimpses of our magnificence and our all-encompassing reality sufficient to know beyond a doubt that we are in fact not a pie made up of separate pieces, but an integrated whole being, resonating with the entire universe. We know deep inside that the part we call "mind" is not separate from another part called "body," which in turn is separate from another part called "spirit." The confusion comes when there is one part or another calling for attention—like when we cut a finger and bleed. In those moments it's clear that the part known as "body" wants some attention. However, as every good mother or father knows, when a child—Sally—cuts her finger she needs a lot more than the best antibiotic cream and designer Band-Aids. She also needs love, reassurance and maybe even a spiritual explanation about why such tragedies as cuts on fingers are permitted in the universe. In other words, even though one aspect of the human being is calling more loudly for attention, the whole person needs to be taken into consideration. Imagine if Sally's dad had to follow all the demarcation rules and first call in an M.D. (He must not touch the finger himself in case his neighbor files suit against him for practicing medicine without a license.) Then a psychotherapist would need to be summoned to help Sally deal with the trauma. (No point in Dad being the possible cause of anxiety for Sally later in life due to a less than perfect therapeutic intervention.) It would then be time to call a preacher to ensure that Sally's spiritual needs were also met. Maybe Dad could buy Sally an ice cream as long as it was low-fat, unsweetened, non-dairy and nutritionally approved. On the other hand, Dad might take a risk and be present to his daughter and her needs by doing his best and getting professional help only when he needed it, as most dads would. It's easy to see that we can become blinded and disempowered by external and self-imposed demarcations of responsibility.

One day one of our Phoenix Rising Yoga therapists called to tell me that she had been verbally attacked by a fellow yoga teacher who appeared threatened by her skills and capacity to serve her clients holistically. He claimed that as a "yoga therapist" she should only work with the physical aspects of yoga and not discuss "that emotional stuff" with them. Her confidence was shaken and she called me for reassurance and reinspiration.

I reminded her of what yoga has been about for the past 4,000 years or so. The yogis did not separate people into bits. In fact, the very word "yoga" means "union." The yogi is concerned with what happens to someone in their body, in their mind and in their spirit and doesn't view those parts separately. It was only when Western medical practitioners went to India and yogis came to the West that a lot of the separation began. Doctors studying yoga in India took their Western analytic models with them. Some Indians, eager to learn from their more affluent and seemingly more astute guests, began to focus more on the development of yoga practices on a medical model. When they tried to determine which specific conditions might be treated with particular techniques, they sometimes lost sight of the other aspects of their tradition.

When yoga came to the West, different yogis focused on different aspects of it. The followers of Paramahansa Yogananda and other teachers like him went deeply into the spiritual aspects of the practice. Meditation was taught and the spiritual elements of yoga were the focus. The concept of transformation and the use of one's life as a transformational tool was paramount.

Around the same time, yoga was also finding its way into America and other Western countries as a pure physical practice. In many cases it was introduced this way to make it palatable to the Western world. Some of the East Indian yogis were very pragmatic. Unattached to tradition, they would do what worked. For several decades in America and some other areas, it has been clear that the Judeo-Christian culture was firmly established and prone to react to any intrusive threat to its spiritual monopoly. In some places, the spiritual aspects of yoga were and still are, seen as such a threat. Many fear that if they practice yoga in all its aspects, particularly the spiritual aspects, they will be competing with established religions. Pragmatic yogis, not wanting to disturb the peace, focused on *hatha* yoga and the spiritual aspects of yoga were downplayed. This approach was more widely accepted than a spiritual approach. As *hatha* yoga became more established, it became known simply as "yoga." If you ask anyone on the street to define yoga you will most likely get an answer that exclusively represents the physicality of the practice.

Yoga with an exclusively physical emphasis becomes a form of exercise somewhat similar to calisthenics. If it is practiced with a competitive- or achievement-oriented motive, it is not that different from any competitive sport. Almost certainly there will be physical benefits from such a practice. To call this yoga, however, sells the practice of yoga short of its potential. If practiced with conscious awareness and as an inner experience as well as a physical form, yoga has the potential to change one's entire life, not just one's body. In his book, *Care of The Soul,* Thomas Moore refers to what he calls "soul yoga" to distinguish between yoga for the soul and the purely physically oriented form of yoga that is more common today in America. To him, "soul yoga" is yoga that serves to open one to an experience of spirit, a way of connecting with the Divine Being that lives within each of us. When our yoga does this for us, it is then yoga in the true sense of the word.

I am often surprised by yoga teachers who faithfully seek out workshop after workshop to learn more and more techniques. Beneath their quest is the belief, "If only I learn enough new techniques to use with my students, I will be a good teacher." Many of them have been practicing for many years and are very adept at guiding their own and their students' bodies into and out of many yoga postures. More postures and more ways of doing them is certainly going to improve their repertoire and enable them to "do" more. But will it serve their students in deepening their practice of yoga? The yoga practitioner or teacher who wants to embrace a soul yoga, or to guide others in a practice that will take them to a deeper level of self-experience, does not need to do much at all. To be successful in this approach to yoga it is more important *how* one chooses to *be* rather than *what* one chooses to *do*.

In training Phoenix Rising Yoga therapists, I often remind students that the most significant thing they bring to the yoga mat when they work with a client is themselves. I also tell them that the being (themselves) they bring to the session is in far better shape if it is empty rather than full of great techniques, ideas and plans. In the early stages of their training they will hear me and believe me intellectually but their old habits will be difficult to shake. They often protest our choice to refrain from giving them a training manual on the first day, and withhold it until after they have completed their first level of training. Our intention is for them to experience the work from the inside out rather than to think it through from the outside in. This is a tough challenge for someone who is used to accumulating knowledge and then figuring out how to use it—and this is the way most of us have been taught to learn. It's amazing how much we miss with this approach. (In learning the deeper aspects of yoga, I would say it is impossible to figure it out with the mind.)

A medical doctor took the first two levels of our training. I admired him for his courage and willingness to put aside his conditioned beliefs and to be a participant in our training program. He had decided to try yoga because of his own experience with an undiagnosed stress-related ailment. After experiencing his first Phoenix Rising Yoga Therapy session he decided to take the training program. The session left him feeling relaxed and at peace with himself and he wanted to learn how to repeat this experience for himself and others. The session worked for him because he had allowed himself, as a client, to be guided through the session and allowed his body to help him let go of his mind.

As soon as he stepped into the training program, however, all his medical school learning habits came to the fore and he became a medical student once again. For most of the first half of the program he sat in sessions with a quizzical, and sometimes puzzled look on his face. During the practical exchange sessions, he was clearly disappointed that his experiences didn't go very deep. Finally, he confided that he didn't fully understand what I was talking about and it was a barrier for him in having a deep experience and in learning the work. He assumed that he first had to understand all of what I was saying before he could have his own experience. I was pleased he was able to acknowledge this, as difficult as it was for him. I invited him to have "any" experience that came to him during the practice exchanges without needing to understand it first, and I told him that we were not asking him to have any particular kind of experience other than his own. Then, afterwards, he could decide what, if anything, he learned from the experience. I empathized with his difficulty in understanding me. I realized how my words would make no sense to him if he expected them to define the kind of experience he was supposed to have, and how to make it happen. I was clearly not delivering those kinds of instructions. My instructions were deliberately vague, so not to get in the way of what was yet to be discovered in the moment.

The other students had not been struggling as much with this process and were operating from a completely different paradigm of learning. I was responding to them and teaching in that same paradigm. To our medical student, it was like being in a foreign country and not knowing the language. When he realized what he was doing, he slowly let go, and by the end of the program was allowing himself to simply be present to his experiences—whatever they were. Frustration gave way to exuberance as he discovered more about himself and allowed himself to be fully present to the experience of each moment. He told us that he was experiencing this for the first time he could remember since childhood. His puzzled look had been replaced by a look of equanimity as he declared to the group, "No matter what, I'm fine just the way I am." He also noticed that the symptoms of his stress-related ailment were no longer manifesting. It's quite amazing how our professions and our skills can sometimes separate us from ourselves in such subtle ways we don't realize it.

I want to be clear that by telling this story I am not in any way denigrating the medical profession or intending to create a "we know but they don't" impression. As I said earlier, the old paradigm has served us well and still does. There is still lots of room in our world for answers. I am not in any way opposed to modern medicine, surgery, aviation, space travel, engineering or any of the professions that use linear thought processes. We need all of them and when we are served by the professionals in any of these fields we will be most comforted in knowing that they have been well trained and do have some answers. If I am flying an airplane and find myself in an emergency situation, I can assure you I will not be attempting to delve into the experience to discover what I can learn. My mind will be searching through my carefully memorized emergency checklist, prepared for the purpose by those who know from previous experience exactly what to do in such a situation. I will trust their knowledge and my memory and resist any temptation to become creative in that moment.

I have discovered that there is more to soul yoga than just the capacity to be in the experience of the moment. The capacity to switch channels from one paradigm to another is also a part of what it's about. I believe paradigm switching will become one of the key skills in our future society. In order to switch paradigms however, one needs to understand which paradigm one is operating within at any given time. This calls for a rather sophisticated level of self-awareness and contextual awareness. I believe the practice of yoga with focused awareness moment-to-moment is one of the best ways we have available for learning this skill. So our yoga will not only nourish our body and soul, it will prepare us for life in the 21st century and a life in which we are continually growing as we open to and learn from all that is happening around us and to us moment-to-moment.

Exercise

GETTING IN TOUCH WITH YOUR SPIRIT

The best way to test some of the concepts in this chapter would be to go and experience a full Phoenix Rising Yoga Therapy session with a trained practitioner. That way you would be able to allow your body to be guided into an experience that would help you get in touch with those other parts of your being, including your spirit. Right now though, you are reading this book, so try this exercise.

Stand at a window and look out. Notice what you see and also notice how you do this. Where do you focus? On what? For how long? Now place your hands on your opposite elbows and make a window frame with your arms. Place your arms on the window ledge and walk back from the window slowly with your legs, letting your head hang between your body and your arms on the window ledge. Notice any discomfort and breathe deeply into it. Hang there for several minutes if you can. Be present to any discomfort, and focus right on it, breathing into it and just "watching" it. Use a deep breath with a focus on the inhale but let the exhaling breath just fall out with no effort at all. Also let the breath make any sounds or noise it wants to. Close your eyes and feel how much you can just let go and surrender into the stretch. Be present to, and stay with the discomfort, but if there is severe pain, stop and come slowly out. After several minutes come slowly up and let your body move in any way it wants to for a little while. Then look out the window again. Notice any difference in the way you are being present to the scene in front of you *now*. What do you notice?

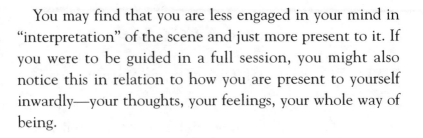 You may find that you are less engaged in your mind in "interpretation" of the scene and just more present to it. If you were to be guided in a full session, you might also notice this in relation to how you are present to yourself inwardly—your thoughts, your feelings, your whole way of being.

10
Tread Softly

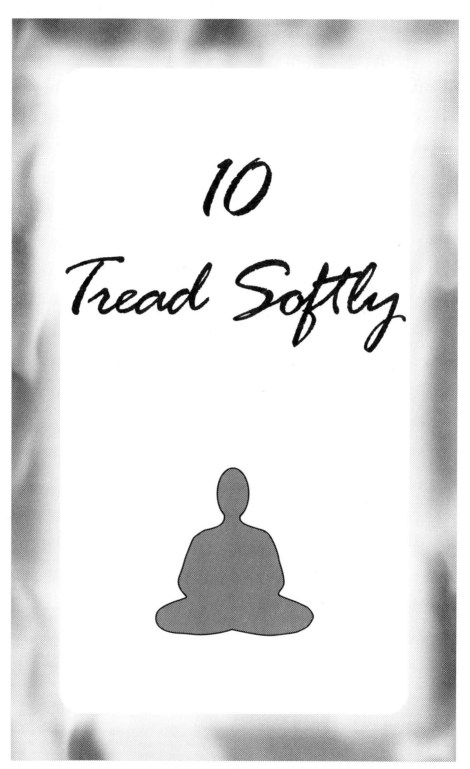

*I*f you practice yoga consciously for long enough, it will change your awareness. You don't even know what it is you are not aware of. Then you become aware and it often seems as if you knew it all the time, except that you didn't.

I remember when I first became aware that my life was, in fact, a journey in spirit. For me, that meant that life wasn't just something that happened to me between birth and death. I had some choice about how to play the game called life. The mere awareness that I had choice meant that my life from that moment was changed forever. Without the knowledge that you have choice, it is easy to live unconsciously. Life can be just something that happens to you. When you know you have choice, it can't. You are then able to decide how to be with it. For me it meant living in a way that brought me into greater harmony with spirit. Ram Dass calls it acting in a way that will relieve suffering, either your own or that of others, and there is really no difference between the two. If you relieve your own suffering, you relieve the suffering of the universe and if you relieve the suffering of someone else, you relieve your own. So I decided to go in that direction, taking care not to make a heavy and righteous trip out of it, which was not easy. I wondered how it would affect my consciousness if I drank beer and ate pizza. Would I not be as well prepared to act consciously in the following hour? If so, should that mean I had better not do it? After this and many other attempts to carefully regulate my moment-to-moment experience of life, I realized I would need to find a way to tread more softly on the path or I would end up with spiritual blight, which I define as ["unable to see the light as a result of working so hard to expel the darkness."]

The awareness that I had during a whole lifetime (and probably many more) in which to do my transformational work helped me tread more softly. There was no hurry. The curriculum was planned by a power greater than I, and the universe would somehow order things in such a way that I would repeat the same lesson until I learned it and the universe didn't care how long it took. All that mattered was that I was willing to be in the school of life with the most honorable intention of taking care of my own and others' suffering as best I could. I would have "on" days and "off" days and the classroom was always there even if I wasn't being fully present 100 percent of the time.

I have discovered that when one is committed to following a purposeful transformational journey in life, there is a process for doing so that can be learned to help soften the road. It's a way of being that we can apply to day-to-day life. It's a skill to be sure, but it's very much like the skill of learning to ride a bicycle. It feels a little awkward at first. In fact it's so awkward that at first we mess it up completely. Later it's just a little wobbly and then later still it begins to feel almost comfortable. Eventually we don't even know we are doing it. It is just a natural way that we live all the time. Although it's possible to learn this process intellectually, it's extremely difficult to apply it with only an intellectual understanding. It's like being trapped in quicksand and trying to read an article on "What to do if trapped in quicksand" to escape. An easier way to learn this valuable process is to use the body as well as the mind.

I think the life process goes like this. First we become aware of some discomfort. This may be reflected physically or emotionally, or it might be a result of our noticing the way we are thinking, or it might be a feeling of a lack of connection (spiritual malaise). We don't know what it is and may be tempted to try hard to figure it out, or alternatively we may witness an old pattern response and cover it up with an escape of some kind. We might be feeling uncomfortable in a relationship, blaming and choosing to avoid the person and the pain. We have done this before. It's a recognizable pattern. At this point, if we have internalized the process well and are no longer simply driven by the first impulse, we step back and sit with whatever it is that is happening. It might seem similar to the following inner dialogue printed with permission from a student's journal:

> *Here I am sitting at home. It's Saturday night and I'm alone. Not only am I alone, I am lonely. I wish there were someone to share my life with. If only I could have had just one successful relationship in my life that lasted. Now I'm paying the price. Maybe I did something awful in a past life to deserve this. Or maybe in this life. Yes, I'm being punished, that is what it is. An empty craving in my gut begins to catch my attention. I feel like sitting down in front of the television with a bottle of something. I want to escape with alcohol and television. It's an old pattern. I have a choice. I can escape if I want. I know it will bring temporary relief. But what about tomorrow, and the next day and the next? What do I really want? What will this experience offer me in the way of transformational opportunity? I don't know. I can't figure it out. So don't try. Just sit with the feelings. Loneliness. Wanting to escape. Wanting something. Wanting to connect. Wanting to matter. Wanting to be valued. Wanting to be nurtured. Wanting to be loved. Wanting all these things. Okay, that's fine. It's okay to want that. What images come to mind when I think of all of that? It comes in the form of one other person. A beautiful woman, being there to provide all that. It's a longing, a craving. And it's here to teach me something. What? Go inside into*

meditation. Look for my Higher Self—the part of me that is beyond the craving. What does it have to say? It's very compassionate and loves me no matter what. It tells me that it really is okay to want what I want. "Give love and you will receive love." Somehow I knew that but had forgotten. As I reflected on the past I could see another pattern. Every time I had let go of my attachment and started to give that which I wanted, I, in fact, received. So what is the next step? Who in my life right now needs my love? With a pen and paper I create a short list. My mom, a friend from work who is recovering from surgery, my ex-wife who is in pain about our daughter's career choice, a colleague who I never have time to talk with but who I know wants to discuss an idea with me. Okay—phone numbers to go with the list and I start dialing. Most of the next three hours is spent listening. By 11 p.m. I am tired, but feeling good inside. I have connected. I feel valued, valuable and loved.

In the above process, Bill chose to accept the awareness that was present and to use it as a tool for learning. You will notice, however, that there was a moment or two of confusion, of not knowing. Bill accepted that, too. He was also open to guidance from within and was willing to try something different—to accept the essence but to change the form. He accepted that he wanted to connect and be loved and loving; he let go of the way in which his mind had set it up to occur in the past and tried something different instead.

Our bodies can teach us this process. If we can practice yoga with conscious awareness, we will learn this process through our body. As we engage a stretch we will come to an edge. This brings us to a moment of choice. There are many ways we can be with that edge. We can run away from it, try to blast through it or just be with it. The last choice is the one that will usually take us further. As we choose to be with our edges in the body, we begin to gain new insights and awareness. Some may be purely physical, but if our awareness runs deep enough, we will begin to see many aspects of ourselves. When these awarenesses arrive, we have yet another choice point. We can accept them or reject them. Again we can run if we want or distract ourselves in some way. Our mind is our most fertile source of distraction. By engaging it externally, we can quickly shut off our awareness of our inner process. To many yoga practitioners, their practice is totally external: "Am I doing the posture right and am I properly aligned?" "Maybe a little more effort and it will look much better," and so on. This kind of focus is not generally supportive of a spiritually transforming experience, nor is it a learning process that can be applied in life. Often it is just a repeat of a well-learned life script that says, "You have got to work hard and you must always get it right and then find a way to do it better."

A greater degree of inner work needs to accompany the practice to make our yoga or our life a transformational experience. It requires being present to all that is happening, internally and externally, as we embrace our edge. It is then necessary for us to take in the experience, whatever it is, with loving acceptance. What we will most likely be called to accept, will be a part of ourselves that is out of balance with our spirit. It may be a frustration calling for a fuller expression of ourselves, a part calling for love, or a hurt part in need of healing and integration. Whatever it is, it offers an opportunity for doing something different than what we may have done in the past, and usually an opportunity to see with new eyes. In order to do this there is a letting go that is required—a leap of faith. It's like standing at the open door of an airplane about to make the first parachute jump. I would feel much more at ease taking the parachute off and sitting back down in my seat than going in this new direction. There is fear of the unknown, a feeling of unfamiliarity and risk.

I recall a lesson that came to me one day in seated forward-bend posture. In this posture you sit with your legs extended forward of your body and straight along the floor. You slowly bend from the hips to allow the upper half of the body to extend forward over the lower half like a jacknife. Most beginners struggle and round their back to force their way down and this can be dangerous to the spine for those with limited flexibility. I had longed to be able to get my forehead out to thumbs which were gripping my toes, but I was a long way short. I noticed when I practiced this posture, how I would have that same feeling of wanting more and being unsatisfied with what was happening. My mind would try to solve my problem and suggest more effort. No matter how much I tried to push past the pain and get further into the posture, I would end up frustrated and even angry. I began to hate this particular posture. And then one day, I saw what was happening. I saw how my mind played itself out every time I was in this posture. Although I instantly wanted to change the script, I had learned enough to know that I must first get to know the old script by watching it even more closely, but from a place of detachment. I did, and I realized how I would often see what "more" needed to happen rather than celebrate "all" that had been done. My focus to improve, to go further, to achieve was good in many ways and had served me in life with the rewards of many accomplishments. At the same time, I often could not turn it off and became angry. I needed to learn how to turn it off and on at will, rather than always being in the mode of "more is better." Over the next several months, the seated forward-bend posture taught me how to do that. I could play with it, sometimes choosing to exert effort and sometimes choosing to let it be fine wherever it was. One day, to my amazement, as I was choosing not to exert effort, I became aware that I was several inches closer to my goal without even trying. I surmised that maybe life could be like that too. It reminded me of my favorite quote by the well-known yogi, B.K.S. Iyengar, from his book, *Light on Yoga:*

> *The person practicing svadhyaya (study/education of the self) reads their own book of life, at the same time that they*

write and revise it. There is a change in one's outlook on life…that all creation is Divine, that there is Divinity within oneself and that the energy which moves one is the same that moves the entire universe.

The good news is that once you have used this process over and over, it begins to become a part of you. It becomes a way of life. You become a continuous happening of transformation. The rough edges of life begin to disappear. The universe no longer needs to send you loud wake-up calls to get your attention. Your attention is more consistently focused on looking at your experiences moment-to-moment and making choices from them that are more in harmony with your true nature. You live your life from a softer place.

Part of this softness, includes your acknowledgment that you are perfect in your imperfections. To successfully follow a transformational path in your life, you must expect to continually become aware of parts of you that are imperfect—places in your life where you have an opportunity to reflect on your way of being and to make a choice about it for the future. Often the revelation of one of these opportunities can be somewhat disturbing.

I recall discovering in my early years of parenting that I often became angry and projected that anger at my children. The awareness was so horrifying that I spent many years in denial about it. Fortunately, one day in a yoga posture, while visiting my "soft place" inside, I got in touch with it. I could feel the fear that was driving my anger. I was saddened by the discovery and I reflected on the many times I had raised my voice in anger and seen the startled look on the faces of my little ones. I had to accept that I was far from perfect. I had to acknowledge that I had been afraid. Afraid of being unable to inspire my children to follow my guidance and frustrated by not knowing how to go about it. Out of my frustration I had tried to power my way through with anger. I also had to acknowledge that at those times with the consciousness and awareness I had, I had done the best I could. Now with new awareness and a willingness to live from a much softer place, I no longer needed or wanted to behave in that way. I had many other options. Feeling guilty would only delay my spiritual journey and would not serve it in any way. It was better to let it go, and get back on the road of life to meet what's coming next, than to stay stuck in self-blame and remorse.

So far so good. Then 10 years later, I again caught myself yelling at my children and it was generated from that same fear. The same old stuff was happening all over again. When this old behavior resurfaces I have at least two choices—pull out the self-flagellation stick and go to work on myself with a sound beating or turn to reflection on what has really happened in those 10 years. I could look at how much I have transformed, taking time to acknowledge how much better my relationships with my children are now and how, on many occasions, I have caught myself about to yell and instead chosen a more mellow and loving mode. I could also support my transformation, and probably that of my children even further by explaining to them that I've just caught myself doing something I don't want to do. I can tell them about the fear that is driving me. They are likely to be much more forgiving of me than I can be of myself and maybe that will help us all a little bit with our collective suffering. For the next few mornings in my yoga practice I can go back to the posture in which I first noticed this fear surface. I can give it the space to surface again if it needs to and allow the opening that occurs in my body in this posture to remind me of the opening coming to me in my life when I am present to my humanity, my fear, my suffering and my capacity to transform it into love.

Exercise

MEDITATION: YOUR BODY AS A GREAT TEACHER

Do this meditation prior to yoga practice.

Close your eyes, focus on the breath coming and going. As you breathe, let your breath bring you in touch with your body. Just allow your breath to connect you with your physical body. As you meet your body, notice anything that might be going through your mind, acknowledge it and then let it go. Simply bring the focus back to the breath and the body. Just the body and the breath.

In meeting your body this day, come to it as you would come to a great teacher. Imagine that you have been seeking someone or something who can impart to you great wisdom—a great teacher. Now I would like you to see your body as that teacher, that source of wisdom. Just as you might come to a great teacher, with that same respect, reverence, and openness to life and discovery. Notice anything that might be in the way of that; any concepts or beliefs that you may have about your body, simply notice them and let them go. Then come again to your body as a wise one. Commit that during your yoga practice today, you will notice your body's urges and feelings and use them to watch your whole self more closely and learn from what you observe. Commit to being soft with the process: "I will use this time to be open, to learn, to experiment. I am soft with myself."

Now come back to the breath, just the breath. Take in a deep breath and let it go with a long, slow exhalation. One more deep breath, and a long, letting-go exhalation. Then come back to your body. Let it move in any way it feels good and then just let your eyes come back open.

11
Perfection

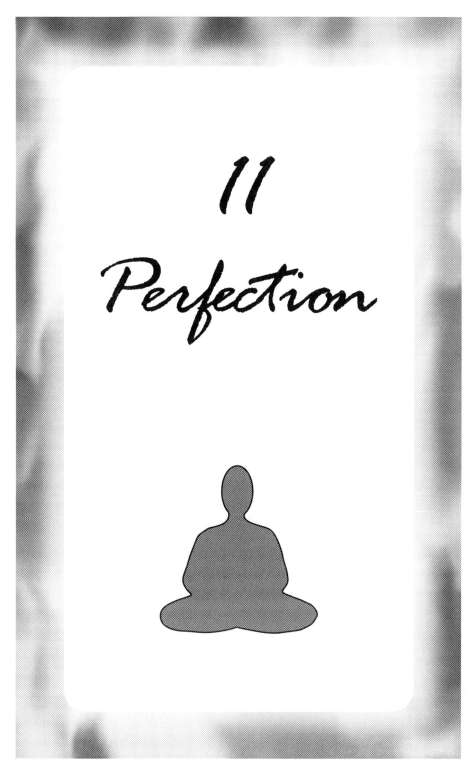

*A*dopting yoga as a lifestyle is a sure way to discover your many imperfections, particularly the physical ones. You will learn the limitations of your body and will be confronted with that awareness. You will either respond in your usual way, or find new responses. You will also notice imperfections in the workings of your mind. Self-doubt, self-criticism, despairing attitudes and beliefs, and even a sense of futility may all arise in your mind's eye. Again you will have choice, to either buy into the script, or to change it.

Being both a spiritual seeker and a human being can create all kinds of dilemmas. Our material world demands perfection on so many levels. In tests at school there is always the possibility of the perfect score. The athlete is often striving for the perfect game. Our technology has made it possible to consistently provide accuracy in calculations. Perfection and the drive for perfection is all around us every day of our lives. If we are not careful, it is easy to become driven by perfection and to then self-reject on the basis of not being perfect or not meeting the impossible standards we set for ourselves. It seems healthy to me to find ways to remind myself that imperfection is, for most of us, a precondition for remaining in human form. If we were perfect, we would have no need to be here in this body and in this classroom called *life*. Life provides us with the opportunities to come face-to-face with those aspects of ourselves that are less evolved and to make choices about them. Simply being present to this possibility means that one is living consciously.

On days when you don't feel like practicing yoga and yet would still like to get in touch with yourself and your world a little more deeply, I highly recommend taking a walk in the woods. Any wooded area will do but the farther away from traffic, other people and buildings the better. I have found being with trees a most wonderful way to connect with my beauty and my ugliness, my healing and my woundedness, my accomplishments and my shame, and most importantly that paradox of life, my perfection and my imperfection occurring in the very same moment.

There is a yoga posture named the tree posture and it's one of the few in Phoenix Rising Yoga Therapy we don't offer as an assisted pose. Trees don't need assistance. They are meant to stand alone. The posture has beautiful imagery connected to it. Stand on one leg, with your other foot tucked into the thigh, and your hands either on the chest in prayer position or raised overhead. Focus on the standing leg and foot to feel groundedness; focus on the uplifted arms to feel the air above. Focus on both to bring them together: "I am the tree. Just like the tree I am perfect in my imperfection. Just like the tree I have my roots in the ground—the earth. I have my arms reaching above to the heavens in a full expression of who I am. I am the tree."

Trees are a great reminder of our uniqueness. They are also a great reminder to take things just the way they are and to appreciate the simple beauty of life. A one-legged yoga posture like the tree posture is very difficult if accompanied by struggle to "get it right," yet much easier when the approach is softer. So often in life we try to make things what they are not—to create struggle—to make something happen that was not meant to be. When we do this, the universe usually lets us know—sometimes gently and sometimes with an abrupt or even painful blow. Often our own agenda for our self-improvement results in our setting impossible tasks for ourselves or tasks that are only possible with great effort and with disastrous side effects. Short-term weight-loss programs are a classic example. We deny our body real food and substitute some chemicals and fluids, thereby inflicting great stress upon our entire organism, all to achieve some desired result conjured up by our mind.

Ted was one of my larger students. In his mid-40s he was well-liked and good-looking but significantly overweight. He was also an irregular attendee at my evening yoga class. Sometimes I would see him every week for six weeks or so and then not see him again for three months. Then he would return for another few weeks and repeat the pattern. Eventually he signed up for yoga therapy sessions and as I got to know him better he told me more about his relationship with his body. He told me how often he would wake up, glance in the mirror and decide it was time to lose 20 pounds. He would leap into action that first day by fasting on fruit and water, then continue to punish himself for five days more to shed the pounds. By day six, he might weigh in seven or eight pounds lighter but couldn't keep up the fruit and water any longer. He would return to a more regular diet but try to be more moderate in his choices. After about 10 days, however, he would lapse and binge on anything and everything. This would be accompanied by intense feelings of guilt and he would go into hiding and avoid socializing for a while. He would eventually return to yoga class because he knew that when he came he felt better about himself. This would last for a while but he would get to a point where he felt the yoga was not working fast enough. He wanted something quicker and more effective to help him trim down. And then he would repeat the cycle all over again.

During several of our sessions we spent a lot of time with me supporting him in an assisted posture while he remained at the edge. I would ask him to tell me about his experience there. When the experience was pleasant he would talk easily about it; whenever it became uncomfortable to him he would not. In integrating one of these experiences he told me that he didn't like to stay very long with anything that either didn't look good or feel good. He would want to brush it aside and move on. In connecting this tendency to his life experience, he realized that he would always only glance at himself in the mirror and would never really look at his body. He didn't really want to see himself. He just wanted to change it. After seeking inner guidance for this issue he told me his homework would be to spend a few minutes each day looking in the mirror at his body, noticing how he felt, and maybe making some new choices about how to see himself. In another session he noticed that when engaging some of the assisted yoga postures he could change his experience of the edge simply by choice. He realized that he could feed his fear of the edge with his mind or he could allow himself into a more loving place from which to experience it. He felt he could do the same thing with his experience of looking at his body in the mirror. Between our sessions, he experimented with this practice and told me how it went.

At first it was difficult. He was aware of his resistance to taking a closer look at his physical body. He allowed himself to experience the resistance and yet still go ahead with the practice. When he began to soften into the edge of noticing his body he noticed it didn't last long. Another edge appeared in the form of self-rejection. Again he was tempted to quit, but again he chose to stay with the practice. In witnessing his discomfort he noticed he could choose how to have the experience. He could do it from a loving place or from a place of judgment and fear. He chose to open his heart to his body and himself and from this loving place the following dialogue emerged and was recorded in his journal.

"Hello body. I know as I look at you I feel judgment, shame and disgust. And I know that my difficulty in accepting you is my difficulty in accepting me. To take the edge off my fear of being with myself, I have used food to help you support me in relieving my pain. You have done that well. You have been a wonderful aid in my cover up. I don't want to do that anymore. I'm now willing to face that pain here on this edge with you. Can you help me with that? In accepting you, I accept me. Together we can change. We can create whatever we want together. Let's try love. I love you, body. I really do."

Ted repeated the practice and the dialogue daily. He began to have deeper experiences in yoga class and in our sessions. He remembered and accepted some early childhood memories of experiencing deep, inner doubts about being accepted and loved by his parents and his brothers. He felt he had never been perfect enough to be really loved. He had tried hard, but always came up short. Eating relieved the pain of trying and failing to be perfect. Now it was time to change all that. He could be imperfect and still be loved, by both himself and others. He wrote in his journal, "I am perfect in my imperfection!"

As in Ted's case, it is not unusual for those using their body as a vehicle for growth, to re-experience early childhood memories. At first I was somewhat skeptical about this. I did not think it was possible. Even when it happened to me and my clients in sessions, I thought perhaps it was a fabrication of the imagination. I am now reasonably certain that in most cases it is not, but is an experience in which some early childhood event or pattern is experienced again. In either case, I believe it can support the transformational process if it is worked with lovingly and consciously and with the focus upon the present and future healing potential, rather than the perils of the past. Unfortunately, there is a tendency to get stuck in anger and blame when traumatic experiences from the past resurface. This does not mean that these feelings should be discounted. Naturally, whatever feelings were activated by the experience need to be honored and felt. That is an essential part of the healing process. It is also an easy place to get stuck. Whatever the experience from the past can offer us in the way of growth, comes from exploring how we might have been choosing to live our lives to protect ourselves from further harm and how we might now choose differently, now that we no longer need to hold that fear from the past. A safe space and time for this transition are important.

I was working with Karen in the seated forward-bend posture. She began to make strange sounds like I had never heard before. The sounds were somewhere between babbling and a baby's cry, and became stronger and louder as we held the posture. As I slowly brought her back out of the posture the sounds changed to a soft whimper with long sighs in between. Back in a prone position on the floor, Karen immediately curled up into the fetal position. I remained with her for several minutes doing nothing other than sitting there with her until the sounds stopped altogether. I then asked her what was happening.

"No one was there," she replied.

"No one was there?"

"Yes, after I was born. . . . I just went back there now to the time just after I was born and I now know what happened."

"You know what happened?"

"Yes. They took me away from my mother. She was very sick. Something happened to her during the birth. So they took me away to a nursery and I didn't get to be with her again for a long time. It was so long I gave up."

"Gave up?"

"Yes. I cried and cried and cried. No one came to me. Crying did not work. So I stopped. I made other sounds instead to comfort myself. I went inside. I checked out. That poor little baby checked out—checked out of life!"

Karen began to cry. This time it was real crying, deep sobbing and wailing. Again, I simply remained focused and present.

When she reached for a tissue and wiped away the tears she laughed. "Wow! That feels so good. That's the first time I think I have ever really cried. You know that?" As she said this she was moving her jaw vigorously from side-to-side. She noticed it, too, and said it felt very different. She had always held her jaw tightly. It had caused her pain from time-to-time in the form of muscle spasms in her neck, throat and jaw. It had not responded well to any treatment she had tried and she had just accepted it as being always there. She said it now felt very loose and pain-free.

In the next 10 minutes, Karen told me more of her story. She had known about her mother's illness at the time of her birth but had not been told, nor had any previous knowledge of a long period of separation. She also could see that there was a significant connection to what she experienced and a pattern in her life. Her prevailing belief had been that there was no point in crying or sharing feelings with anyone because no one would be there anyway and she would just show up as imperfect with all her wounds. In times of emotional need the only thing to do was to withdraw inwardly and comfort herself the best she could. She had never been able to cry. Somehow her jaw would not function in a way that would allow it to happen. She explained how the strange sound was a way that she used to take the crying inside rather than let it out. When she made that sound she could feel it in her chest and belly and it was her way of comforting herself. She now had a new experience. She had let the cry out and had felt better. Maybe she could let the cry out more often. Maybe her pain was worthy of being experienced rather than being hidden inside. It did not matter if anyone noticed or not. Her cry was for herself. Her birth experience had made her different. If she acknowledged it, she saw herself as imperfect. Now being imperfect, with those feelings, was acceptable. There was perfection in letting what was true for her be fully experienced. In so being, the pain lost its power.

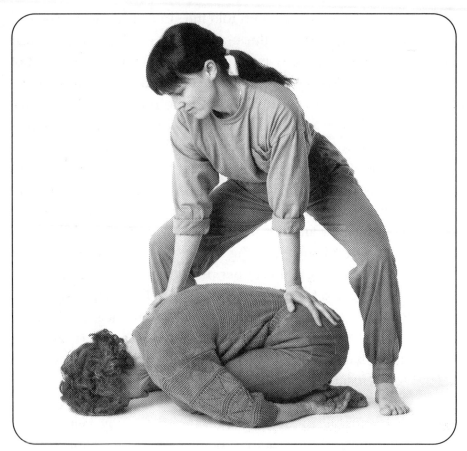

The child's pose

Exercise

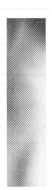

GOING BACK TO THE WOMB

Curl up on the floor like a baby in the womb with your head tucked into your knees which are drawn up to your belly. Spend a few minutes taking deep full breaths and experience your body fully. Let your awareness take you back to being in the same position in your mother's womb. What was it like there? What was happening on the outside? Were you ready to be born or would you have preferred to stay in the womb? What was the family and the world like that you were born into? What fears do you think this little baby had to deal with? And how did he/she do that?

Next, let your body respond to this question. Let it flow into whatever spontaneous movements or positions feel right for it. What do these body postures express? What is your body saying and how is it trying to move you in life right now?

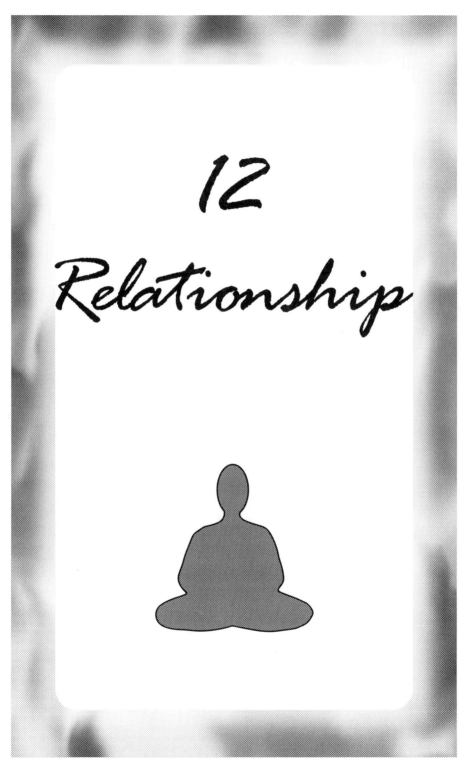

12
Relationship

*Y*oga helps us to examine our relationships. Particularly our relationships with ourselves, which of course is a barometer for our relationships with others.

One morning after my yoga and meditation practice, I was feeling very connected and was in deep reflection. I thought about myself in relation to others and quickly reviewed my most significant relationships with others. As if in a flash of momentary insight I saw how *all* these relationships and their depth of intimacy were of my own creation.

I repeated to myself in awe, "I *have* the relationships that I have created." I was surprised. I had probably played intellectually with that concept before, but this time I was not only thinking it, but feeling it and really knowing it to be true. There, in that moment, I was accepting total responsibility for the health of all the relationships in my life. I know that when I am truly spiritually empowered—that is, when I am living from my spirit and not from either my reaction to things or my concepts about how things are, or should be—I am also choosing how to be present with all that exists around me and selecting what works for my spiritual nourishment and what doesn't. I must say that I do not live from this place all the time. Far from it. Most of the time I am living from concepts and sometimes from reaction.

I look back at my relationship with my wife, Lori. For 10 years we have lived as husband and wife; we run a business together, we have two children, and we are both individually and collectively very effective at manifesting in the world and in living from our spirits. What bewilders me about myself in this relationship is that during the first seven of these 10 years, I resisted commitment. Even with all the yoga I had done, all the growing that I had done and all the fears I had explored, I had managed to hold back for seven years on becoming legally married. I rationalized my choice with thoughts like, "It really doesn't matter," and "It's only a legal 'thing'—we are spiritually married anyway." In more honest moments, I may have come a little closer to the truth by saying, "I was married to my first wife for 17 years and felt that I had been deeply hurt so let's just keep things as they are and not risk that again. Why risk spoiling a good thing?"

What was really happening? I was afraid—that's what. Afraid at a very deep level that I could not create the relationship I wanted. That may appear contradictory because for seven years, I had a great relationship. Yes, we had our moments when I had my doubts and she had hers, and we did things that were hurtful to each other at times, but when I was connected to my source, I was clear that this was a relationship that I wanted. It was also a relationship that was serving me well by enhancing my spiritual growth—something I also believe important. Whenever we would practice yoga together, we would sometimes sit across from each other in meditation and I would experience a level of bliss that far transcends that excitement one feels in the primary arousal stage of a relationship. After those moments we would sometimes verbally affirm our deep inner feelings, and I would *know* without doubt that this person sitting across from me was here to teach me and that our being together was a source of food for my soul. And still I resisted commitment and even did things that would put the relationship at risk. Why?

I had believed that my first marriage was a special one, too, and I had been deeply hurt. If I could create the relationship I wanted, how come I couldn't do it there? What chance was there that I could do it now? On further reflection now, I see that I could have created it there, too, but again there was resistance. I had been more wedded to my beliefs and fears in those days than to a fellow human being. The way I reacted to circumstances around me often prevented me from a deeper connection to my truth. I spent more time in *reaction* than in *creative action*. How easy it is to do that.

My first wife and I married very young. We were both just 22 years old. To me, at that time, she was the most beautiful person I had met. I remember a fearful voice inside me asking, "What if I never find anyone else as beautiful as she?" My response was, "Maybe I had better get married to prevent that from happening." My young mind had found a solution to my fear rather than an answer from my soul. Many years later I was to learn that fear-based solutions in response to issues that arise in relationships, are wonderful ways to set up karmic lessons. Anything you do to get what you want from another that comes primarily from your fear, will sooner or later come back to bite you if you stay in that relationship. And so it was with my first wife. The thing I feared the most and set up to prevent was the very thing that happened 17 years later. She left. Did I create that in this relationship? I believe I did in a subtle way. I was probably pushing her away for many years, in a metaphysical sense, and would have known this had I been aware enough to see it.

I do not blame myself for my lack of awareness. I was where I was. And given my state of awareness, this was probably the only way for the relationship to go. I had committed to it from a place of fear and unless I had been able to see that and willing to re-establish the basis for the relationship, it clearly could not have endured.

I began to become more aware of what was happening as a direct outcome of my daily yoga practice and the awarenesses that came to me via my body in moments of deep, inner connection. As I began to attune more deeply to my whole being through my practice, I would experience occasional insights into who I was and who I was becoming. I began to see how many of my decisions in earlier years had been based on fear. Not the deep kind of fear that stops you in your tracks, but rather the kind of fear that says, "You might never be able to get what you really want so grab what you can if, and when, it appears."

I gradually began to accept responsibility for the way in which I had created and was maintaining the relationship.

In a healthy relationship, we are doing that all the time. We are checking in with our spirit and rediscovering what is true for us. In a healthy relationship, we are looking for opportunities to grow and ways to bring the level of communication with our partner to an even deeper level of truth. In a true spiritual relationship, we are taking care of our own growth and noticing how our partner contributes to that. We are seeing where our blocks are and we communicate them. When we see collusion or codependence with our partner stemming from our mutual areas of unconsciousness, we are careful to explore them in the context of our deep love for each other rather than blaming the other for also being imperfect. We are willing to risk being honest about how it is, for the sake of our continuing growth. We are each, at times, the teacher for the other and the student of the other. We are the mirror for each other.

Often we don't know the answers. We can only feel the pain. These are often hard places to *be*. We get very tempted to start *doing* and trying to *know* or taking the seemingly easier option of running away. When the mind is engaged in its unique version of righteousness it is difficult to disengage from it long enough to check in with one's spirit. Again, however, our body can be a beautiful ally if we choose to use it as such. It is indeed the gateway to our spirit and a far more reliable instrument than the mind in times of such crises. Our body is a friend that will rarely let us down, anytime we want to find the way "home."

When I find myself "getting off the rails" with my partner I will often take a time-out to get present to myself first before inviting her to support my commitment to a clearing between us. It may mean doing a little yoga and meditation or just going for a walk alone. I will then invite her to share a brief attunement with me. It may mean just sitting quietly together. Sometimes it may be in the same room, or on occasions when the sparks have been really flying we may require a little more distance and need to spend a little time meditating alone. Inevitably, during this time we will each independently get a glimpse of where we have been withholding our love from each other, or denying our resistance. We will each begin a process of softening. Then from this softer place we are ready to begin to dialogue and talk not from righteousness but from our commitment to our truth, and to each other. Often this will involve each of us revealing our fears and some of those dark areas within us that are yet to be transformed. This supports an opening to each other as we recognize our "stuck" places in ourselves and each other and at the same time catch a glimpse of the majesty of spirit working through our humanness. We are in love once again. In love with ourselves and with each other. No matter how hard I try, I find it almost impossible to begin this process with my mind, particularly when I am upset. I need to disengage my mind, go to my body, and let it take me to that place inside that is beyond the turmoil. Then I can find the love again, which I may have temporarily lost.

I have seen many times how I hold the power to create the outcome I desire in my relationships. The outcome I refer to is not necessarily getting what I want or the other person getting what she wants. There is something in relationships much deeper that just our surface wants. It is the state of love that can exist between two beings when they are both in their truth and experiencing each other's Divinity as well as their humanness. To do this, my first and most fundamental task is to begin with myself. If ever I find myself out of relationship with anyone I must first discover what is happening for me in that relationship. That means searching for my "stuff" exclusively. What is it that is happening here that I am reacting to? Can I be the witness to myself and see where I am stuck? What is it that I am unwilling to let go of? I personally find I can do this far better when I use my body and my practice of yoga to soften away the rough edges that are present around my wanting to be right and blame the other. If I am not in a place to let go of these rough edges, then the chances of any fruitful dialogue occurring between me and the other person are slim. I am most likely to slide into reaction, which in turn will probably result in the other reacting and the fight will continue. If I can *own* my part of what is really happening, it will be so much easier for the other to do likewise. Then if I can truly listen as the other shares about herself without reacting, even if it does drift into blaming me here and there, then we may be on the way to moving it to a state of grace. Sometimes it's possible to listen through the blame to the place where the hurt is coming from, and from this level of understanding and empathy the other is most likely to also soften.

I see the relationship between client and Phoenix Rising Yoga therapist as a relationship model from which I draw much inspiration for all of my other relationships. The therapist learns to be present in a certain way. With experience this learning is internalized to the extent that it has become a natural state of being—being 100 percent present, open, out of the way, a loving mirror reflecting the wisdom, the power and the love emerging from the soul of the client. It is a magical relationship and has on many occasions brought me to tears as I sit in awe of the beauty of it as it unfolds. In the early stages of learning, before this way of being present is fully internalized and has become a natural state, we have to consistently make the choice to be present in this way. We have to watch ourselves and remind ourselves to come back to loving presence when we lose it. We could, if we chose, do this in all of our relationships most of the time—an awesome possibility.

Recently, I returned home from a teaching assignment and I came into our office to see a new high-quality scanner sitting next to the main computer. I knew Lori had been wanting one for some time to add better quality to our printed materials and advertisements. When I saw it, I had mixed feelings. I knew it was a piece of equipment that would be great for our office but I was annoyed that I had not been consulted on the decision to buy it, given my job of balancing our budget. My first reaction was to go to Lori and demand, "How come you bought that damned thing while I was away?" thereby, putting her on the spot to explain herself. I sensed I was more furious than I first thought and it was time for a deeper check-in with myself before saying anything. I went into my office, calmed my mind with some deep breaths and a five-minute meditation, did some stretches to open up my chest and feel my heart, then sat again and waited for guidance from within. It said, "Don't react. Just listen with love. All will be well if you stay non-reactive and listen."

I found Lori, saw her through loving eyes and saw the joy in her eyes, took some more breaths, and said with as much love as I could generate, "Hey, I noticed the new scanner and would love you to tell me more about it and your decision to buy it." After listening to all the wonderful thoughts that had gone on in her process to obtain this new tool, she also volunteered, "And you know, I wasn't sure if I should wait to tell you about it before I bought it. I know it's a big purchase and something you would probably want to be in on, so I'm so pleased you are not upset about it. I knew you would want to check out our cash flow first, so I did that before I ordered it!" (Wow . . . did she ever know me well?) This gave me the opportunity to share my truth. I told her that at first I did feel hurt about being left out of the decision but had chosen not to react and that now I was pleased to hear how excited she was and how responsibly she had considered the decision. I had let go of my hurt as I had listened to her. She was touched by my honesty, my decision not to react and my openness and she was now hearing me deeply as well. This led to the creation of one of those magical moments of taking each other in and having the experience of love that comes from it. It also had given me a chance to let go of my fears and reach a deeper level of trust. I notice that every time I'm able to do this it gets easier. At the same time, I notice that there are still times when I don't get to this place of consciousness and react in my old way instead. When that happens, I notice it, forgive myself and take corrective action. I am learning and I give myself full permission to be a learner, to stumble and fall, and sometimes feel the excitement of taking a few steps in the direction I want to go in creating the relationships I want in my life.

I also have to admit it's a lot more difficult to choose to shift your way of being in close relationships than it is in a session with a client or in the classroom. In a session, you are with a client that you don't live with. Once the session is over, they are out the door and on with their life and you are on with yours. There is no attachment on your part to any adjustment happening. With your family or partner, there is often such an attachment. You want the relationship to work out and you would prefer the other person did the adjusting to make that happen. So part of making the shift to showing up differently in your relationships also involves letting go of your attachments, or at least recognizing them and choosing to put them on the shelf for a while. Yoga offers a great vehicle for seeing your attachments. And once you see them, they are released more easily.

When I walk in the door of my house after a long trip away, I notice that I have many attachments and many choices. I can choose which ones to take with me into the house. I could walk in with, "What's been happening here while I've been away?" (Investigative mode.) Or I could try, "I've had a long hard trip and need to be taken care of." (Little boy mode.) Another option, and the one that I prefer is, "I'm so pleased to be home and want to take each of you in and feel your presence. I also want to appreciate you and our home." (Grateful joy mode.) I recently got to the door with my grateful joy mode all in place to find nobody home. Ah well, take a few breaths, be present in my body, and celebrate yet another opportunity to release attachment and find grateful joy with my house plants and the clothes in my closet as I unpack my bag. Today, I am home, inside and out. Thank you, God.

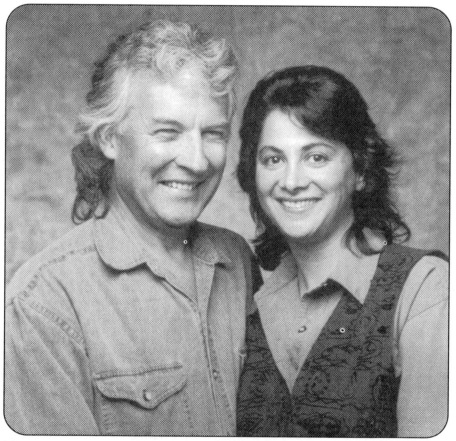

Michael Lee and his wife and partner, Lori Bashour.

Exercise

DISCOVERING YOUR SOUL ATTRACTION TO YOUR PARTNER

Sit on the floor in a cross-legged position with your partner sitting opposite and your knees touching. Take a few moments to close your eyes and breathe. Center yourself in your own body and at the same time be aware of your partner's presence. Then open your eyes and sit in silence while focusing your gaze on the point midway between your partner's eyes. Hold that position and that gaze for several minutes without talking or making any facial expression. Continue to breathe deeply and easily. Just be together without needing to do anything or respond in any way.

Take a few extra moments to get in touch with your partner's "essence." What is it about this person at the deepest possible level—the soul level—that you find yourself drawn to?

Verbally share with each other what that is. Tell each other what this experience of relating in this way was like for you.

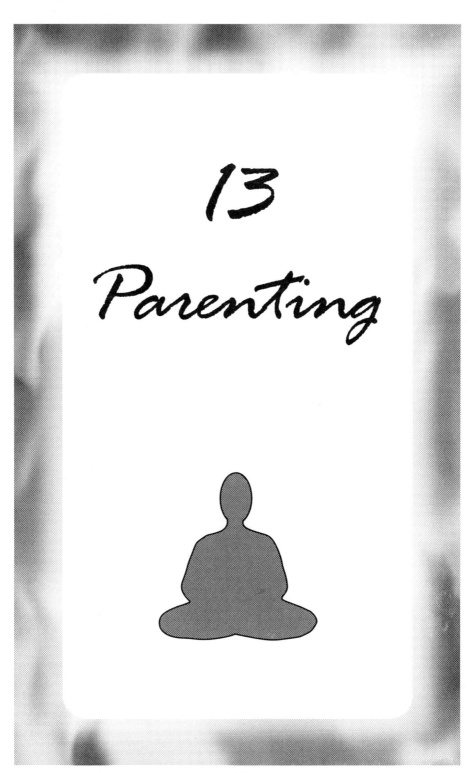

13
Parenting

*W*hen you think about it, being a parent is very much like a 90-minute strenuous yoga routine, only expanded into 20 years or more. You come up against all kinds of edges, find numerous opportunities of choosing how to be present with what is happening, and find out a lot about yourself in the process. I believe yoga can help us tremendously in meeting the challenge of parenting in the 21st century.

I also believe that parenting in the 21st century is very different from any other time in history. Only 50 or so years ago, we could almost predict that things would not change a lot from one generation to another. Not so now. When I grew up in Australia, I did not see television until I was 11 years old. Now just 40 years later, my children learned to navigate their way around the Internet long before age 10. Children of today no longer believe that the education system can teach them a finite body of knowledge that will equip them for life. They understand the need to learn how to learn and how to access information as a solid foundation in any education. By the time they become teenagers, they are probably much more adept at accessing information about anything, than both parents combined. Old systems of control, used for generations of parenting, no longer apply. How can you control someone who has more information about everything than you do? It's a set-up for failure. Instead, parents must learn how to be enrollers and know how to inspire their offspring into playing a game of life that works and offers results worth achieving. They also have to provide the safety of structure and boundaries that used to once be provided by society at large, but which now no longer exist. They have to do this in the face of uncertainty and with inadequate training for the job. It makes parenting a much more difficult and more daunting task than ever before, but one that if handled well, will continue to speed up the incredible transformation of consciousness that is accompanying the technological revolution. It takes some focused commitment, though, to get there.

I remember when my first-born child was in her mid- to late teens. I was a single parent struggling to raise a teenage daughter and her younger brother. By this time, I had developed a daily yoga practice and used it as my anchor to life. My daughter was pressing up against every boundary I had established. In hindsight, my boundaries were probably way too tight. I was scared. She was my only daughter. I didn't want any harm to come to her. I'm sure the story is a familiar one. I was being an overprotective dad and it clearly wasn't working. She was being a rebellious and somewhat troubled teenager. I didn't know which way to turn. Each morning in my yoga practice I would try to let go of the worry. Trying didn't work. In fact, it has been said that when you are trying to do something you are not really doing it—and I was clearly not doing it. It was during those moments that I sometimes doubted the effectiveness of my yoga practice. My mind would engage thoughts like, "How come I can't let go of this problem?" and "What good is my yoga practice if I get calm in the morning and then become a worried, angry, over-controlling dad by early afternoon, when I find my daughter has skipped school again?"

One morning in my practice I realized I was truly not trying. Maybe I had let go of trying or given up—I'm not sure which. I had begun a new routine involving lots of standing postures. One posture was *garurasana*—the eagle pose. This is a somewhat difficult balance posture, which involves balancing on one leg with the other leg intertwined around the standing leg. The arms are intertwined with the hands in front of the face. The gaze, like that of an eagle, is focused directly ahead.

As I practiced I thought about my daughter. If only I could figure out how to "fix" the problems she was having and everything would come back to "normal." Of course I never could. I entered the eagle posture. I had to concentrate to hold my balance and my mind shifted focus from my daughter to the balance in the posture. Once established in the posture I began to experience the feelings and images associated with being an eagle—spiritual vision, a reserve of power to be used wisely and only if needed, balance, one pointedness, deep concentration, gazing into the sun with an elevated clarity. I affirmed to myself "I am the eagle!"

Thoughts of my daughter returned but I remained in the energy of the eagle. As the eagle, I saw myself giving my little eagle (my daughter) more space to experience her own wings, and trusting that she would learn, and that even if she crashed, there was very little I could do now anyway. It is said that the eagle has incredibly powerful eyesight and that it can look directly into the sun—symbolizing looking directly at the Father (the masculine aspect of the Divine). I was beginning to experience the power and the trust of that Divine Father.

That afternoon I sat down with her and told her that I could no longer take responsibility for the outcome of her life and had learned that I must now give that to her. I told her I cared for her and loved her, told her she now had to make choices in life for herself (which she was doing anyway), and that I would always be there if she needed my support or counsel. From that day on, we became more comfortable both in our relationship and in our shared day-to-day lives. In my parenting, from that day forth, I took the eagle with me, into my being. It remains with me and is a part of who I am as a parent.

Years later, on reflection, I see that it's not so much what I *do* as a parent that matters as much as how I *be*. When I am being a father with the qualities I deem important in fathering, then my parenting takes on a whole new dimension and becomes a relatively easy role. When I try to plot and plan with my mind about what I should do, without dropping into a state of who I am, or who I want to be as a parent, I struggle in the role.

My daughter was not only instrumental in teaching me about parenting. She also had the honor of teaching me my first lessons in the yoga of grandparenting as the following extract from my journal illustrates.

Becoming a grandpa for the first time gives me much to think about. Twenty-five years earlier I was a father for the first time. And here I am, still a work in progress, still struggling with all those life issues like relationships, responsibility, accountability, integrity and so forth. I'm an unfinished grandpa. And that's a surprise. After all, weren't grandpas supposed to have it all together? Be wise and all-knowing? And here I am, a grandpa, still hard at work on my own dharmic evolution. And despite my "unfinishedness" and my hit-and-miss parenting of my dear daughter and her three brothers, she has not only survived but has actually nourished the growth of the family tree by giving birth to little Robert. All I can say is, "Wow!"

As an aspiring yogi, I have to take a little time out and see if there is not something more to learn from this new posture of "Grandpaness." For years now, I've been teaching my yoga therapy clients and students to "be in the experience," "breathe into the posture" and "see what it has to teach you." I believe what we learn on the yoga mat has application to life, and then how we approach the postures in life can also be learning experiences. The yoga posture is life in miniature. The big postures happen in life day-to-day. Like becoming grandpa. So what can I learn from this posture?

First, my daughter calls me and says she is going to be

having her baby in two days and would be having her labor induced. She also tells me she will be given medication during labor to minimize the pain. I immediately go into an internal reaction. Luckily, I pick up on my body signals enough to recognize the reaction and not launch into a spontaneous lecture on natural childbirth. After all, 25 years ago her mother and I had sweat it out with a natural birth. We had compromised on going to a hospital rather than having a home birth, but insisted it be totally natural and drug-free. Now here was the result of that 20-hour labor, my daughter, now choosing differently. What sort of a yogi was I to have created this? I take one breath, catch what my mind is doing, process it, integrate it and let it go—all in two seconds flat. Then I utter, "That's wonderful, Dear, I'll be there."

Off the phone, I ask myself: "What have I done? How can I leave all the things I have to do, the rest of my family, and head off to somewhere in Georgia for four days? Does that make sense? Of course it doesn't, but something inside says, 'Go!'" So, I did.

Next afternoon, bouncing around in an airplane in turbulence on my way to Atlanta, I have time to do a little more processing and meditation. "Let go, let go," comes the inner voice. "This is not your call. Step back, Grandpa. Your role is different here. It's time to learn the distinction between doing and being. The distinction between being a parent and being a grandparent. Parents do, grandparents be. Your job is to be present in this posture. That's all." Haaaa! Another deep breath. I'm engaging the posture.

I arrive at Keiron's home, connect with her and her husband again, place my hand on her belly and feel the baby's movements and experience the excitement of the impending birth. I'm in the posture taking in that first sweet feeling of bliss. All is well.

Next morning, Keiron leaves early for the hospital to begin the induction. I arrive a few hours later and she is in labor. Nothing to do but be present. Focus and wait. A few hours pass, contractions are stronger, she asks for, and receives, pain medication. I take another deep breath. Now I'm really in the posture and experiencing some discomfort. Breathe and let go. Haaaaaa!

My son-in-law, Bob, happens to be working on a construction site right at the hospital. How convenient. But today he is not working but being present with Keiron for the birth of his son. This part of the posture feels good. "Aaaaaah." Bob wants to go over to the construction site, just minutes away to see his father and brothers and tell them what's happening. He asks me if I want to go. Keiron's Mom is there with her and a little break in the action would be good. I go along. We put on our hard hats and hang out for a few minutes with the men at the site. We talk about the impending birth from that cool, detached, no big deal, kind of place that only men on a construction site could. Bob's beeper makes some noise. He looks at it and breaks away in a fast gallop back to the hospital with me in hot pursuit. It's Keiron, letting him know that it's time to return as "something's happening." My heart beats faster; the posture is getting intense.

We rush into the delivery room to Keiron's side, still wearing hard hats. The nurse present and Keiron's mom crack-up in amusement. Light relief. Keep breathing though, you are still in the posture. "Aaaaaah."

My grandson is ready to be born. We are only waiting for a doctor. "Why?" I ask. "Is he necessary?" Ooops....Don't interfere....I almost fell out of the posture. Back in....Breathe...."Aaah."

Keiron asks for the lights to be dimmed and for her favorite chanting tape, "Lady Mass," to be played. "Ahhhh."...How sweet. How beautifully spiritual. Those two years she lived in an ashram had some effect. Ooops….More mind-chatter. Back to the posture. Be present. Be present. Breathe.

Doctor arrives in traditional hospital ritual fashion. My mind avoids comment. I'm doing better. He adopts his position and tells Keiron it's okay to push. Three pushes later and voilà… little Bob is born.

We all cry. The tears for me are tears of joy and also tears of deep bliss from once again experiencing the miracle of birth. A new life, a spirit takes body form and enters the world. And I am his grandpa. How awesome. I like this posture. I really can let go into it now and come out of it feeling its benefits. I have been touched by the grace of God, once more. Being here was the right choice. Thank you, God.

Exercise

A YOGA POSTURE FOR PARENTS: THE EAGLE

As with many yoga postures, the way into the eagle posture is critical. If we don't focus on this part of the posture, it often doesn't happen. Begin with deep full breaths and a sense of freedom though the body. Take a deep breath and on the exhale intertwine the arms and hands, right under left. Focus on the right leg which will be the standing or supporting leg. Slightly bend it at the knee, and keeping the focus on its support, on another exhaling breath, lift the left thigh high up over the right and lace the left foot behind the right calf. Lengthen the whole body slightly and open the chest and throat. If you fall out of the posture, take a deep breath and start again from the very beginning, taking your time. Once established in the posture, focus your gaze on a spot directly in front and breathe deeply. Become the eagle—focused, aware, present, ever-watching, strong. Affirm, "I am the eagle."

14

Independence

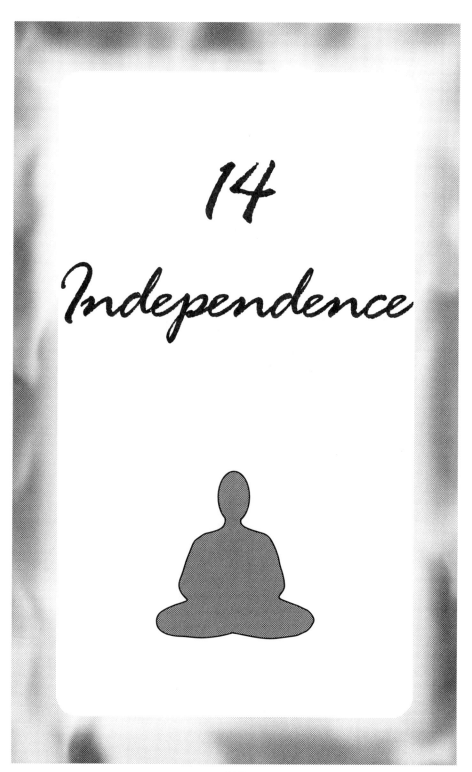

*W*hether we like it or not, one inescapable reality is that as long as we inhabit a human body we must live in the world around us. Yes, there are many forms of escape available, both internal and external, but those of us reading this book are probably convinced that such escapes offer only short-term results and long-term pain if we overuse them. So we must take our place in the world and take a stand for life. As with all aspects of life, I believe the practice of yoga offers much to us in terms of supporting our level of comfort in the world, especially in this emerging age of information and technology. Basically though, the lessons for life are much the same as they have always been. We just need to use the skills with a little more frequency and finesse.

Every fourth of July we celebrate Independence Day. What we are celebrating is really a very significant event in the evolution of our nation. We are celebrating a time when as a community of people, we decided to stand on our own two feet, a time to no longer be subservient, a time to accept responsibility for taking this stand in shaping our own destiny. What our forebearers did collectively back then as a political action, we each are called to do in our own lives at some time. Perhaps there are many occasions in our lives when we are required to take a stand for something important or something we strongly believe. Sometimes we do it well and sometimes not. Taking a stand on anything requires courage, clarity, focus, commitment and self-expression. For many of us, such qualities need to be developed and strengthened. Our yoga practice can help us.

I remember one of my early yoga classes: standing bow pose; me wobbling all over the place; trying to focus my eyes on a spot on the wall to maintain balance; teacher talking to me—"Michael, how do you think you can stand on your own two feet when you can't even stand on one foot?" That didn't help my balance very much and I was also quite puzzled. Maybe I was missing something—surely standing on one foot was more difficult than standing on two. "What was he talking about? Hate this posture. Can't wait for the next." Wobble, wobble. "Damn posture!"

Some years later while practicing the same posture, the light went on. I got it! By working with the posture and learning about it (and of course about me as well, including my fear of maturing/growing up), I discovered that one of the secrets of all standing postures is where to put one's focus. Sure, it helps to look at a spot on the wall to focus attention, but where in my body should the focus be? I had discovered that if I could plant my focus firmly into my standing leg, visualizing it as a firm, strong, straight support, it would do its job and hold me in position while the rest of the posture happened above. That standing leg was my base, my rock of support. Also in life, we need to take care of our base (or our basics) before we can do much else. We need to firmly direct our focus to our source of support, acknowledge it, feel it, enjoy it, and then move out from it, trusting its ongoing presence. Without it we are on shaky ground and will find ourselves without the platform needed for artful self-expression. Wobble, wobble.

I also noticed over the years of practicing the standing bow, and other one-legged standing poses, that strengthening each leg in turn as we do, gave me a different sense of myself while standing on two legs. By learning how to support myself on one leg, it was so much easier to stand firmly on two, especially when focusing on both. I began to see a little of what my teacher had meant about being able to stand on one leg as a step towards being able to stand on two.

I also noticed the inner shifts that came with such a practice: more confidence, a greater capacity to take a stand in life with less fear of being knocked over, a greater willingness to challenge that which needs to be challenged and the strength to endure whatever results from that. It's indeed a powerful posture for life enhancement and maturity and a way of learning independence and being able to stand on my own two feet.

Standing on our own two feet in the new world we live in is becoming an increasingly complex task for many. Old ways of doing things are becoming redundant almost as quickly as last month's newest computer. Simply learning what we need to learn to master the new technology in our lives is often an awesome task. There is no doubt in my mind that the practice of yoga and the acquired inner disciplines that come with consistent and deep practice, facilitate our capacity to learn new things and to adapt to a changing environment. When I came to live at Kripalu in 1984, I knew little about computers and could not type unless I painstakingly used two fingers. Studying part time, I decided to learn keyboarding skills and also a little about computers. My next-door neighbor had one of the early Apple computers and offered to let me use it and to borrow a typing tutorial program. At this time, I was also practicing up to four hours of yoga per day. I was surprised at the speed with which I found my way around the computer and also learned to type. Within a few months I was turning out my college work in print with relative ease. I noticed how I could focus and how my brain *and* body (particularly my fingers) would "remember" things. I had once tried to learn to type in my 20s and gave up as a failure. Now I was learning effortlessly as long as I took the time to focus on the sequenced tutorials. I was amazed but not surprised. My time on the yoga mat was directly supporting my capacity to focus and to learn.

Some years later I began to see the same process at work with many of my clients and students. It seemed those who could learn the art of using the external yoga posture as a way of developing inner focus, could transfer this capacity to many life situations. During the summers when we had a yoga studio in Stockbridge, Massachusetts. I was invited to lead some yoga workshops for the students participating in the Jazz Dance Program at Jacob's Pillow, a summer dance theatre company. These students were young, athletic, flexible and talented. They appeared to be very comfortable in their bodies and I really doubted if there was much I could teach them. I was surprised at what happened. After I had guided them in some partner work using inner-focusing techniques and holding several postures at their edge while engaging some inner dialogue, I saw many of them change their physical appearance and seem to enter a deep, internal state. In the discussion that followed, some students spoke about really "tuning in" to their bodies for the first time and developing a more acute awareness of their whole being. Two of them later told me how having such an experience had permanently enhanced their dance performances from that day on.

In the last few years of this millennium, we are seeing an upsurge in the popularity of the age-old practice of yoga to the extent that it has become mainstream. This is unparalleled in modern history. The practice is most likely more popular now than it was in any of the previous six thousand years of its history. Why?

To begin with I think there is the "baby boom" effect. Most "boomers" were around in the 1960s when the Beatles went off to spend time with the Maharishi. The Beatles showed their generation and the world that there may be something of intrinsic value in the mysterious practices of the East. That wasn't enough however, to turn a generation of boomers into yogis, although for a number of years throughout the '60s, '70s and '80s, there was a fairly steady migration of Eastern yogis to Western shores and they all had little difficulty in developing a following. But that is nothing compared to what is happening today. Gurus from the East seem now to be waning in their popularity but the practice of yoga is still booming.

The first boomers have hit 50-plus and their health and longevity have become more important than ever before. And apart from its esoteric appeal, yoga has some very clear health benefits. It improves the circulation and the functioning of glands and organs, tones the body, enhances respiration and you just plain "feel better." There are many practitioners who practice solely for these physical benefits and there are many teachers who provide that focus. Like everything American, yoga in America today comes in a variety of forms ranging from the more traditional Eastern mystical focus to a pure western physical "macho" focus with brand names like "Power Yoga."

Regardless of the form, however, all the modern practices have some link to the ancient traditions—otherwise why call it yoga? I believe that it is this connection to a deeper source, despite the waning of the gurus, that has as much to do with the growing popularity of the practice as it does the obvious physical benefits. Sure, we want to take care of our physical well-being, and for many it is worth spending an hour or so a day to get into our bodies and work out, be it yoga, weightlifting or jogging. But that's not all. The society we are creating at this time in the history of humankind has certain features that make it ripe for a practice like yoga to take root and flourish.

Our technological and information age has provided many benefits and in many ways has simplified our life. On the other hand, it has also made life more complex. In the last half of the 20th century, we have probably been called upon to make more adjustments in any given life span than any previous generations have been called to do. We have to adjust to changing relationships between the sexes, environmental concerns, new ways of doing business, a changing economy, related employment issues and so forth. Living easily in such a world often calls for large adjustments in one's state of being internally as well as externally.

Those who are unable to adjust may not become extinct right away like the dinosaurs, but they will most certainly experience a lot of stress in their lives. It is likely that the more difficult the adjustments, the greater the stress. Those who are in touch with their state of being at a deeper level and are able to rapidly process new ideas and the associated feelings and then reflect the changes in new external behavior more appropriate to the situation, are much less likely to experience stress in the long run. A healthy body that is used as a vehicle to enter deeper levels of awareness is a tool that is almost essential to such a way of being. I believe this is why we are seeing such a tremendous upsurge of interest in the body/mind connection in the fields of well-care and health education and why practices like yoga have become so popular in recent years.

If practiced with focused awareness and an attitude of loving acceptance as it is in a Phoenix Rising session, yoga has the potential to provide many more benefits to enhance the already apparent physical ones.

Mental clarity is one of them. Our minds are very busy these days. The input into our brain on a daily basis is enormous. More likely, it's more information than any brain can really process. But it tries. It's not surprising that such mental overload can lead to confusion and even despair.

If we can focus on our body and attune to it, and at the same time let our mind free-wheel, it might slow it down and help it get a sharper focus. We will then be better equipped to face each new day and the mental challenges it presents.

Emotional stability is also a quality in high demand these days. Linked to our fast pace of life, we are often unable to process our experiences of life adequately or deal effectively with the emotional components of these experiences. We begin to ride the emotional rollercoaster leaping from one emotional state to another. We become a victim to our emotions rather than using them for the purpose of greater life understanding and effectiveness. Again, yoga can, and does, help. It can provide a time-out to take our feelings a little deeper and with greater acceptance of them. We can breathe into our feelings and give them space, and so begin to feel a little more at ease with ourselves and our lives.

Spiritual attunement is more than likely the benefit most sought after by the early yogis and most often overlooked by the modern yogi of today. Yet when a glimpse of it is derived from one's yoga practice, we come back for more. It makes sense as it is surely an element missing for most of us in our lives to some degree. What is it? To define it simply, I would say it's about being in touch with ourselves and our universe. We get some sense of knowing what we are here for. Or at least some understanding that being here in this body and in this life is part of something bigger than us, and that it's perfectly right, just the way it is. So much for simple definitions. Anyway, however you define it, my guess is that greater spiritual attunement is possible for the yoga practitioner of today who wants it.

As Phoenix Rising Yoga therapists, our intention has been to create a way for yoga to provide people with an opportunity to receive all of these life-enhancing benefits, should they want them. In our sessions, the client is guided through their body, to a deeper experience of all aspects of themselves on many levels. They also reap the physical benefits of enhanced circulation, respiration and body functioning; and develop greater mental clarity, emotional stability and spiritual attunement. In an integration phase, they also connect their yoga experience to their life experience so that each day they can apply their new awareness to produce a fuller and more joyous life, in harmony with spirit. Yoga practiced in this way is clearly a life-enhancing activity. And when we have it, we want more.

Because of this, I am certain that the art of yoga in general and adaptations like Phoenix Rising Yoga Therapy, will continue to increase in popularity in our world in the foreseeable future. It will continue to provide many with the vehicle they need to live more independently and effectively in a rapidly changing world.

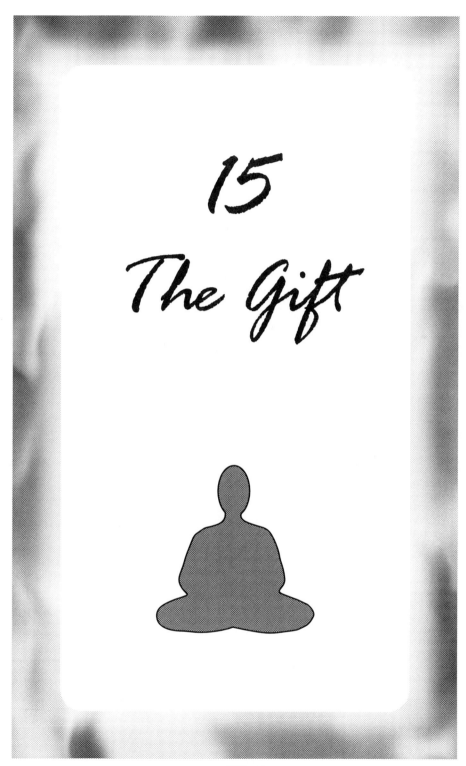

15

The Gift

*W*e all have at least one gift available to us to use in this life. Our gift usually comes to us early and then stays with us throughout our life. For example, the gift of persuasion possessed by those who are able to sell either material goods or ideas to others, is often possessed by those who learned at a tender young age to use this skill to get their needs met by the significant adults in their life at that time. Like all gifts, it usually comes from something we learn to do well in order to get what we need or want. It works for us and so we continue to use it.

Cynthia was a marathon runner. She was also a mother of three children, and since returning to her profession as an interior decorator had, in the space of three years, grown her home-based business to provide her with a good income. Her husband was also successful in his career and the time they shared together, although not abundant, was generally pleasant and enjoyable. The children were well-cared for with a schedule that would impress a Swiss railroad manager. Approaching her 40th birthday, Cynthia began to notice that her body was not supporting her as well as it always had. She was in good health but often felt tired and slow in the mornings and didn't seem to have the stamina and endurance she previously had. She also began to notice a soreness in her muscles that seemed to last longer than usual. A friend suggested she come with her to her yoga class. At first, Cynthia resisted, thinking that yoga was not for someone like her. She didn't like the idea of moving slowly and being still. Cynthia saw herself as a woman of action who needed to move. Yoga did not seem like something she would enjoy. For some reason though, maybe because as a runner she appreciated the value of stretching or maybe just to humor her friend, she went to her first yoga class.

The class was led by Laurie, a practicing Phoenix Rising Yoga therapist and yoga teacher. Laurie was not quite what Cynthia had expected. She was vibrant, funny, down-to-earth and welcoming. It didn't take Cynthia long to feel comfortable and to get into the energy of the class. She liked the brisk warm-up exercises and the breathing exercises. Laurie's careful guidance into each posture and her subtle invitation to her class to focus on their total experience with acceptance rather than striving to reach some imaginary goal, made it easy for Cynthia, yet demanded her presence and focus. By the end of her first class, she could feel the benefits. She felt lighter, more expansive and more vibrant. She felt good. Noticing that Laurie also offered one-on-one Phoenix Rising Yoga Therapy sessions, Cynthia decided to try that as well and received weekly sessions from Laurie over the following three months.

During one of those sessions, as she focused on the sensations in her chest while in an assisted posture Laurie was supporting, she had several flashes of herself as a little girl. They all involved her success in achieving results. Whenever she completed a difficult task or reached some important goal, her parents were pleased and she received love, affection and praise. In the integration part of the session she was able to connect some of these childhood experiences to her life and to acknowledge her incredible capacity to make things happen, to run marathons, to train long hours, to organize and plan, and generally live a very focused and productive life. She was both aware of and grateful for this gift.

In a subsequent session, while attending to the feelings in her belly, another memory surfaced. She was in college and a member of the Student Politics Club. She was in a group meeting to organize a campus political rally to cover some important issue. She felt very strongly about the particular aspect of the issue to be discussed and wanted to be one of the speakers at the rally. Although she could speak well enough in public, she knew that others in the group were much more experienced for that particular role. She could either speak up at the meeting and offer herself as a speaker and risk rejection or remain silent. Neither option appealed. In the next few moments someone suggested that they would also need someone to volunteer to organize all the logistics and equipment and make all the arrangements with the school office for the rally. Seizing her opportunity, Cynthia volunteered herself. It gave her a way to contribute, and to be recognized and accepted for getting a job done. At the same time she could feel the empty feeling in her belly that was caused by her disappointment in not being one of the speakers.

In integrating this session, she saw how the same pattern was present in her life today. She relied on her gift of being able to get things done to win her acceptance in her family. It was relatively easy. She was a good organizer, producer and achiever. Deep down though, she experienced a feeling in her belly from time-to-time when she wanted things to be different. There was a Cynthia who wanted the freedom to express some of her more outrageous thoughts. Many times she had wanted to go to town meetings and school board meetings and say her piece without fear of the consequences. Most often though, she had opted to serve on the various support committees and leave the talking to someone else. She now saw that her gift was also a source of limitation. The gift had a shadow and hiding in it was perhaps another gift yet to be discovered.

Over the course of the next year, Cynthia continued her yoga practice, her business and her running. She also became politically active in her local community and in her professional association. She was at first concerned that she would not have sufficient time for all of it but didn't let the concern stop her. Instead, she created more time for herself by hiring someone to help her with the production tasks in her business. This led to her confronting the uncomfortable feeling that no one else could do it as well as she had. After all, she was a gifted producer and it would be extremely difficult for anyone to even approach her standard. Going deeper into these feelings however, Cynthia saw how being a great producer had protected her from the awful feeling of being unimportant and possibly unloved—the worst possibility of all.

Every time she spoke up at town meetings Cynthia feared such an outcome. Many times she felt like running rather than speaking. To her surprise, she oftentimes had more supporters than opponents. She also noticed the change in the sensations in her body in those moments as she took more risks. It felt more alive and she felt more passionate about life and everything in it. Although busier than ever before, her interactions with her husband and her children seemed to be deeper and more meaningful. As her life became richer and more colorful, so did theirs. There were adjustment conflicts along the way from time-to-time but there was no turning back and they all knew it. Cynthia was emerging from the shadow of her gift and discovering two gifts instead of one.

I love telling Cynthia's story because it illustrates the possibility of transformation in the life of someone who already had a successful life. Transformation does not often come easy to such people. There is no great incentive to change and often a fear of upsetting something that is already good. The old expression, "If it ain't broke don't fix it," often applies. I believe that such people are often well-served by a body-oriented approach to transformation, as Cynthia was. The body is a useful tool to bypass the mind that wants to keep things just the way they are. Often, though, the mind will resist any attempt to use the body in such a way. It almost happened for Cynthia. She didn't think yoga was for her. It was too slow and not sufficiently fast-moving. Keeping the body moving at a fast pace is a great way to ignore its deeper messages. Endurance athletes are often highly skilled at engaging their bodies in a battle with their mind.

The strength of mind forces the body into superhuman tasks. On one hand, this is a gift. On the other hand, it often prevents seeing what hides in the shadow of the gift.

This is where a practice such as yoga can be greatly beneficial, although it too can be used as a battleground between mind and body. Many yoga practitioners practice with the mindset of an endurance athlete with a focus on achievement. If getting results and accomplishing feats in life is not something they have already learned to do well, then such a practice is possibly highly beneficial. The body can be used to teach the value of achievement. If, however, such an approach is merely a replay of an already mastered skill in other areas of life, it is not of great transformational value. The practitioner would be better served by going to a class like the one described here or receiving individual sessions like those Laurie gave Cynthia. Laurie had the skill of being able to facilitate a body experience for Cynthia that took her out of the achievement mode and into a mode of deep, inner listening. She became aware of feelings and sensations in her body, possibly for the first time. When she tuned into these she saw both her gift and how with overuse it prevented another part of her from coming forth. There was of course a price to pay for such awareness. She had to challenge her old and comfortable ways of being and risk showing up without praise and a feeling of being loved. There was also the need to pass on her gift to another who was less accomplished, giving that person an opportunity to learn as well.

Cynthia's story also illustrates how the wave of transformation extends beyond the person embracing change. Her relationship with her family changed, as did her place in her community and among her colleagues. In a sometimes subtle way and other times more directly, this created the opportunity for all of these people to show up differently in their world even if only in minuscule ways. In finding a way to integrate the new gift Cynthia was allowing to come forth, they too would have an opportunity to transform. Such change might also be accompanied by resistance and reaction but even this could be the fuel for transformation in the future. I recall hearing someone once say that one of the ways to transform our world is to begin by transforming ourselves. I now see, years later, the wisdom in those words. By freeing ourselves sufficiently to allow more of our gifts to come out of our shadows, we create beautiful ripples of transformation going out in all directions.

Exercise

New Ways of Being

Meditate quietly for a few moments without thought and then ask this question of yourself: "What is my gift in life?" Continue to ask and listen until you receive a clear indication of what it might be. Then ask, "How does my gift limit me and prevent me from needing to learn in life?" Again continue to ask the question until clarity comes. Then ask the third question, "What opportunity in learning is here for me and how do I want to approach it?" Journal your responses. Now read your responses and as you do, check into your body. Visualize and sense your body posture in situations where you are using your gift. Do the same for those moments when you overuse your gift. Visualize and sense a scene in which you are learning a new way of being without overusing your gift. Notice what happens in your body. Over the next month stay aware of the times you use your gift, overuse your gift and try new ways of being. Notice the accompanying body sensations on each occasion.

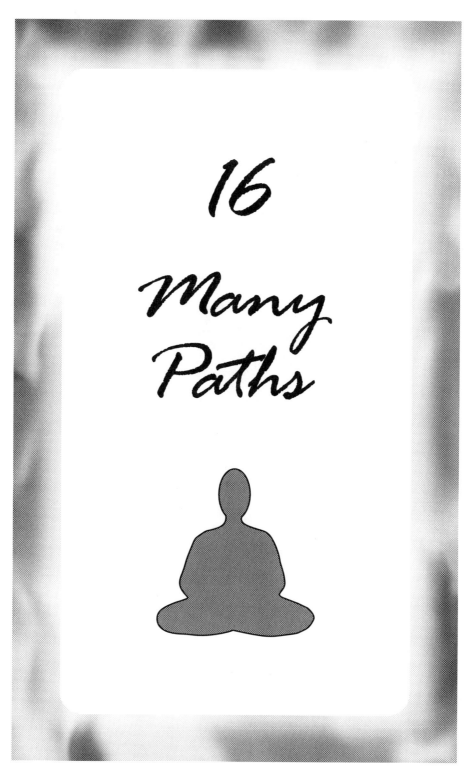

16

Many Paths

*I*t's been said before and I believe it is true, "There are many paths to the mountain top." In terms of the technology for transformation, there are many teachers, many ways to transform, many paths. Different paths and different teachers emphasize different aspects and use different methods. Some are suitable for certain people depending on what they might be needing at that time to support their journey. In the order of the universe, there are no "wrong" choices. We are all going to the same place anyway, no matter what route we take to get there. Even if we do nothing and are unconscious of the transformation process, we will still transform—like it or not. Life will still present us with food for our soul. We may choose not to digest or even recognize it, but it will keep on coming no matter what.

Given that there are no wrong choices, then does it matter much what one does? Will any path suffice? Will any teacher provide the lessons we need? The answer to these questions is ultimately, "yes." In the short run and from a practical perspective, however, there may be a shortcut to the process. Why take a lifetime to learn what might be available in a few days or even a few hours? On the other hand, why hurry? We may prefer to enjoy the ride rather than travel hastily to the destination.

We were doing a weekend workshop in Banff, Canada, one of the most beautiful places on earth in any season. It happened to be winter and there was a few feet of new powder snow all around. We wanted to be out in it. I had learned to cross-country ski only a few years

earlier, having come from Australia where it was not a widely practiced sport. I had developed my skills to the extent that I could get
along well on the flat terrain and could handle moderate terrain
going downhill with reasonable conditions and gentle turns. My
assistant and good friend Lee had never skied before but wanted to
try. Being an always-willing teacher, I told him I would help him
learn. We rented equipment and headed out. We put our skis on at
the trail head and, following the few pointers I gave him on tech-
nique, Lee seemed able to move along the flat pathway with relative
ease. Anxious to go, he asked, "Where does the trail begin?"
I pointed to an opening in a wooden fence slightly downhill from
where we were standing and said, "Right there." Lee dug his poles
into the snow and headed for the designated opening. He gained
speed, veered slightly off course, missed the opening and wrapped
himself and his skis around the fence, going over it head first and
landing on the other side. In an instant, I realized there was a lot
more to teaching Lee to ski than I had first thought. I felt badly for
not being a good teacher, apologized, helped him to his feet and
suggested we go back to the lodge and find a better instructor.

It was clear to me that there were things that a good teacher could
teach Lee and maybe save him some trouble at the outset. With me
as his teacher, he might learn to ski eventually but it would be
mostly by trial-and-error and only marginally better than teaching
himself. I was surprised, therefore, when he resisted my suggestion of
getting a more qualified instructor.

"We can do this," he said. "I've learned a lot already. Just show me
how to stop and how to turn."

"But Lee, just now I forgot to mention turning and stopping and
you went into a fence. Wouldn't you feel more comfortable with a
better teacher?" I asked.

"No, I'll just be a little less ambitious and ask you what I need to
know and it will work out fine. Besides, we are on the other side of
the fence now anyway," he said.

We laughed and had a lot of fun for the next few hours, by which time Lee was skiing as well as he wanted to, for a first time out.

This story really says a lot more about Lee than it does about learning to ski. Lee had done a lot of work on himself over his years of practicing and teaching yoga. He was very confident in his capacity to learn and even more importantly, he wanted to take responsibility for his own learning. He knew that it would be easier for him to do that with me with no lesson plan than with an instructor with a clear step-by-step agenda. Like a well-accomplished student, Lee trusted he could find out what he wanted to learn and leave what he didn't, even with this new skill. He could surrender to receiving the wisdom of someone else when he needed to. It wasn't just his ego that prompted his desire to be responsible for his own learning. He was able to make that a choice and go either way. He either needed to have an expert show him or not. Either way was fine, depending on the circumstances. Such a student is empowered. Such a student needs a teacher who will support empowerment. Such a teacher is often not easy to find. Many teachers are attached to their lesson plans, attached to being the expert, and limited to a one-way power-relationship that says, "I know—you don't," and, "I teach—you learn."

Clearly, on this beautiful day in Banff, Lee was opting for an easier method of education, even if it was a little less precise.

The same is true for anyone wanting to learn more about the game of life; use their body as a vehicle and yoga as a practice. Teachers come in many different forms. There are many different aspects of yoga and all teachers will have a particular preference. Better educated students make for better teachers. If you're looking for a teacher, it's important to ask yourself, "what am I looking for?" particularly in terms of results. Do you want a body/mind experience of yoga or just a physical experience until you learn more? Do you want to be challenged, and if so, to what extent? Do you want a teacher you can relate to or just someone who knows what to tell you to do? Just like shopping for clothes, there is nothing wrong with trying on several different styles and teachers.

In training Phoenix Rising Yoga therapists and teachers, we focus on those aspects that we consider important. From my own experience in transformation through yoga, I felt the greatest breakthroughs when I was free to do my own inner work which needed to come from the inside out. I wanted someone there who could support me physically in the postures, maybe ask a few opening questions, but largely leave me to create my own inner dialogue and determine what, if any, significance it held for my life. I didn't want to be diagnosed, interpreted or counseled. As a result of these preferences, we have trained practitioners who will be totally present to their clients, but who also know how to be out of the way and allow the client to do their own work. In order for one to get to this place, however, there are some things you have to know, so we also train our practitioners to educate their clients about how to receive the work. They need to be able to recognize the things they need to be responsible for and what they need to have the client be responsible for. It's an edge and sometimes there can be confusion, but with training it is a learnable and an effective way to work. There are, however, many clients unfamiliar with, and not ready for, this kind of approach. They demand an expert and require that expert to control and direct not only the process but also the outcome. I don't believe it's possible for me to do that for anyone in the game of life as each life is different, requiring its own unique approach which can only come from within each of us. Since I don't know what is resonating within you, the best I can do is create and guide a process that will help you discover it for yourself.

So, although there are many paths to the mountain top there are also many paths with dead-ends. Beware of anyone who offers to relieve you of the responsibility of finding your own path and your own unique answers to your major life questions. The relief of not needing to do your own work, will probably be temporary and may even be a distraction. In the game of life, I suggest seeking teachers who will teach you how to find your own answers rather than give you answers. The same applies to practices and process work you engage in. Look for practices that may not have short-term results and, over time, can support you in developing your own inner knowing.

Many practices of Eastern origin that have come to the West have come along with attached rituals and many cultural trappings. Some yoga teachers insist on using the Sanskrit names for yoga postures. While there is much to be said for this practice in that it supports deeper understanding if one is familiar with some of the language, it is not essential. The same applies to the wearing of certain clothes or colors. While there is no doubt some spiritual significance for such preferences, they are again peripheral to the essence of the practice and not a prerequisite for spiritual growth. On the other hand, some students react so strongly to certain preferences of their teachers, that they disregard their entire offering merely because they don't like the way they dress, or the language they use. This also can be a mistake. Both students and teachers need to look beyond the superficial and ask the more important questions. For students it might be, "Is there something valuable about me, and for the game of life, that I can learn through this person?" For teachers, it could be, "How can I deliver the essence of what I am here to teach without getting caught up in the costuming of it?"

I have also learned that the best teachers are often those who are not attached to keeping their students, but who celebrate when it is time for the student to graduate and move on. In the game of life we need students to become teachers who can, in turn, empower other students. A good teacher is also one who celebrates her students arriving at some place in their evolution that far exceeds her own knowing, just as a wise parent celebrates when his children evolve their awareness beyond his.

It is an exciting time that we live in as we enter the third millennium. Technological advances have brought us to a crossroads at which one of the choices presented to us is to follow the inner path as a way of continuing our collective evolution. It is an attractive path right now. Many of us long for a regeneration of our spirit connection. We are also well-positioned to take it. There are many vehicles and many teachers. Wise choices, together with a firm but not inflexible commitment will take many of us to new levels of awareness from which to serve ourselves and others. May your journey be bountiful.

Phoenix Rising Yoga Therapy Resources

Yoga Tape

A 45-minute yoga class led by author Michael Lee entitled "Yoga—It's About Life." Suited for beginners and experienced yoga students, the cassette tape presents an easy-to-follow yoga experience which incorporates many of the principles outlined in this book. Side B contains a short lecture by Michael Lee about how to integrate yoga into your daily life. Cost: $12.50 plus shipping and handling. Call (800) 288-9642.

Therapist Certification Training Program

For information about becoming a Phoenix Rising practitioner or learning more about how this exciting modality can enhance your existing career call (800) 288-9642 or e-mail: PRYTOFF@aol.com or check out the Phoenix Rising web site at: www.pryt.com.

Informational Video

A 30-minute video tape about the Phoenix Rising Yoga Therapy training program. The video is informational, not instructional. Cost: $10.00. VHS format. Call (800) 288-9642.

Referrals

There are more than 800 trained Phoenix Rising Yoga practitioners worldwide. If you would like to receive information about a one-on-one session (fees vary) with a practitioner in your area, call (413) 274-6166.

Schedule of Phoenix Rising Yoga Programs

To receive a schedule of programs and workshops led by Michael Lee and other trained Phoenix Rising workshop leaders, call (800) 288-9642.

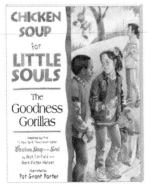
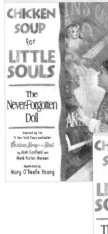
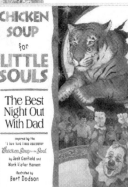
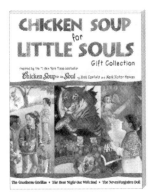